Facial Injuries in Sports

Editor

MICHAEL J. STUART

CLINICS IN
SPORTS MEDICINE

www.sportsmed.theclinics.com

Consulting Editor
MARK D. MILLER

April 2017 • Volume 36 • Number 2

ELSEVIER

1600 John F. Kennedy Boulevard • Suite 1800 • Philadelphia, Pennsylvania, 19103-2899

http://www.theclinics.com

CLINICS IN SPORTS MEDICINE Volume 36, Number 2
April 2017 ISSN 0278-5919, ISBN-13: 978-0-323-52431-5

Editor: Lauren Boyle
Developmental Editor: Donald Mumford

Clinics in Sports Medicine (ISSN 0278-5919) is published quarterly by Elsevier Inc., 360 Park Avenue South, New York, NY 10010-1710. Months of issue are January, April, July, and October. Business and Editorial Offices: 1600 John F. Kennedy Blvd., Ste. 1800, Philadelphia, PA 19103-2899. Customer Service Office: 3251 Riverport Lane, Maryland Heights, MO 63043. Periodicals postage paid at New York, NY and additional mailing offices. Subscription prices are $343.00 per year (US individuals), $627.00 per year (US institutions), $100.00 per year (US students), $389.00 per year (Canadian individuals), $774.00 per year (Canadian institutions), $235.00 (Canadian students), $475.00 per year (foreign individuals), $774.00 per year (foreign institutions), and $235.00 per year (foreign students). Foreign air speed delivery is included in all *Clinics* subscription prices. All prices are subject to change without notice. **POSTMASTER:** Send address changes to *Clinics in Sports Medicine*, Elsevier Health Sciences Division, Subscription Customer Service, 3251 Riverport Lane, Maryland Heights, MO 63043. Customer Service (orders, claims, online, change of address): Elsevier Health Sciences Division, Subscription Customer Service, 3251 Riverport Lane, Maryland Heights, MO 63043. **Tel: 1-800-654-2452 (U.S. and Canada); 314-447-8871 (outside U.S. and Canada). Fax: 314-447-8029. E-mail: journalscustomerservice-usa@elsevier.com (for print support); journalsonlinesupport-usa@ elsevier.com (for online support).**

Reprints. For copies of 100 or more of articles in this publication, please contact the Commercial Reprints Department, Elsevier Inc., 360 Park Avenue South, New York, NY 10010-1710. Tel.: 212-633-3874; Fax: 212-633-3820; E-mail: reprints@elsevier.com.

Clinics in Sports Medicine is covered in *MEDLINE/PubMed (Index Medicus) Current Contents/Clinical Medicine, Excerpta Medica,* and *ISI/Biomed.*

Contributors

CONSULTING EDITOR

MARK D. MILLER, MD
S. Ward Casscells Professor, Head, Division of Sports Medicine, Department of Orthopaedic Surgery, University of Virginia, Charlottesville, Virginia; Team Physician, James Madison University, Harrisonburg, Virginia

EDITOR

MICHAEL J. STUART, MD
Professor, Department of Orthopedics, Chair, Division of Sports Medicine, Mayo Clinic, Rochester, Minnesota

AUTHORS

AMANDA M. BLACK, CAT(C), MSc
Sport Injury Prevention Research Centre, Faculty of Kinesiology, University of Calgary, Hotchkiss Brain Institute, Cumming School of Medicine, University of Calgary, Alberta Children's Hospital Research Institute, Cumming School of Medicine, University of Calgary, Calgary, Alberta, Canada

MATTHEW L. CARLSON, MD
Department of Otorhinolaryngology, Mayo Clinic, Rochester, Minnesota

ANTHONY CLOUGH, BDS (Hons LON)
Scientific Committee Member, Medical Commission – Games Group, International Olympic Committee, Lausanne, Switzerland; Dental Advisor, GB Boxing, Lecturer, Oral Health Essex University, Lecturer, Sports Dentistry, Eastman Dental Institute, University College London, London, United Kingdom

KRISTI COLBENSON, MD
Consultant and Assistant Program Director, Emergency Medicine, Consultant, Sports Medicine, Mayo Clinic, Rochester, Minnesota

MICHAEL EASTERBROOK, MD, FRCSC, FACS
Department of Ophthalmology and Vision Sciences, University of Toronto, Toronto, Ontario, Canada

PAUL H. ELIASON, MSc
Sport Injury Prevention Research Centre, Faculty of Kinesiology, University of Calgary, Hotchkiss Brain Institute, Cumming School of Medicine, University of Calgary, Alberta Children's Hospital Research Institute, Cumming School of Medicine, University of Calgary, Calgary, Alberta, Canada

CAROLYN A. EMERY, PT, PhD
Sport Injury Prevention Research Centre, Faculty of Kinesiology, University of Calgary, Hotchkiss Brain Institute, Cumming School of Medicine, University of Calgary, Alberta Children's Hospital Research Institute, Cumming School of Medicine, University of Calgary, Departments of Pediatrics and Community Health Sciences, Cumming School of Medicine, University of Calgary, Calgary, Alberta, Canada

GRANT S. HAMILTON III, MD
Assistant Professor, Department of Otorhinolaryngology, Mayo Clinic, Rochester, Minnesota

GUY L. LANZI, DMD
Attending Physician, Department of Surgery, Cooper University Hospital, Camden, New Jersey

ALEXANDER P. MARSTON, MD
Resident Physician, Department of Otorhinolaryngology, Mayo Clinic, Rochester, Minnesota

JONATHAN A. MICIELI, MD, CM
Department of Ophthalmology and Vision Sciences, University of Toronto, Toronto, Ontario, Canada

ERIN K. O'BRIEN, MD
Assistant Professor, Department of Otorhinolaryngology, Mayo Clinic, Rochester, Minnesota

L. MARIEL OSETINSKY, MD
Department of Otorhinolaryngology, Mayo Clinic, Rochester, Minnesota

RAY PADILLA, DDS
Faculty, School of Dentistry, University of California, Los Angeles, Team Dentist of Athletics, University of California, Los Angeles, Team Dentist, Los Angeles Lakers, Team Dentist, Los Angeles Galaxy, Los Angeles, California

DECLAN A. PATTON, PhD
Sport Injury Prevention Research Centre, Faculty of Kinesiology, University of Calgary, Hotchkiss Brain Institute, Cumming School of Medicine, University of Calgary, Alberta Children's Hospital Research Institute, Cumming School of Medicine, University of Calgary, Calgary, Alberta, Canada; Australian Collaboration for Research into Injury in Sport and Its Prevention (ACRISP), Federation University, Ballarat, Victoria, Australia

GABRIELLA PICCININNI, BS
Science, Technology and Society, Stanford University, Stanford, California; Medical Services Coordinator, World U20 Hockey Championship, IIHF, Toronto

PAUL PICCININNI, BSc, DDS
Dental Expert Member, Medical Commission – Games Group, International Olympic Committee, Lausanne, Switzerland; Member, Medical Committee, International Ice Hockey Federation, Zurich, Switzerland; Team Dentist, Mississauga Steelheads, Canadian Hockey League, Mississauga, Ontario, Canada

CHRISTOPHER F. VIOZZI, DDS, MD
Assistant Professor of Surgery, Mayo Clinic, Rochester, Minnesota

Contents

Facial injuries can pose a large health burden for athletes, potentially resulting in time loss and surgery. This article reviews the incidence, common mechanisms, and risk factors of facial injuries in several sports globally. Estimates of facial injury rates are complicated by a lack of, or inconsistent, reporting on specific types of injury. Much of the epidemiologic literature is based on hospital-based injury surveillance and there is a paucity of literature examining sport-specific risk factors. Future research should focus on prospective injury surveillance methodologies with consistent injury definitions examining risk factors and the effectiveness of facial injury prevention efforts.

There is evidence that eye protection, mouth guards, helmets, and face guards are effective in reducing the risk of facial injury; however, such safety practices are not adopted universally by all athletes playing high-risk sports. Underlying beliefs about risk perception, comfort, ineffectiveness, utility, and a lack of awareness or enforcement have been identified as reasons people may not adopt preventive measures. There are several high-risk sports that have not mandated or do not enforce use of protective equipment. Valid evidence can assist with addressing the resistance caused by prevailing beliefs and could be essential in influencing rule changes.

On-the-field evaluation of facial trauma requires a focused initial assessment of the patient's airway and breathing with a knowledge of the critical associated injuries. The initial triage in facial trauma involves assessing and protecting the athlete's airway, breathing, and cervical spine. The algorithm then requires a repeat evaluation for subtle causes of airway obstruction and aspiration risks. Final steps include control of hemorrhage, recognition of neurologic and ophthalmologic disability, and complete exposure of the athlete to examine for other associated injury. The

ABC repeat ABCDE mnemonic allows providers to avoid missing critical injuries that require immediate intervention.

This article reviews the diagnosis and treatment of facial soft tissue injuries in athletics. General diagnostic algorithms are presented, including initial assessment aligned with Advanced Trauma Life Support guidelines. Specific injury types are discussed along with possible collateral damage and adverse sequelae to limit morbidity. Treatment modalities are described using generally accepted principles refined to fit athlete patients. Return-to-play issues are outlined relative to level of participation, with the emphasis on safe return. Goals of treatment are defined, including prompt, accurate diagnosis; efficient, effective treatment; safe return; and optimum functional and esthetic outcome.

Sports-related eye and orbital injuries continue to occur regularly and may have serious consequences. They are completely preventable when appropriate protection is worn, particularly with polycarbonate lenses. Eye protection is available for most sports and should be worn in accordance with the standards of regional authorities. It is important for first responders to identify red flags in the history and physical examination of an injured athlete for urgent referral to an ophthalmologist. Common sports-related eye injuries include corneal abrasion, subconjunctival hemorrhage, hyphema, vitreous hemorrhage, retinal tears and detachment. The mechanism and treatment of these injuries are discussed in further detail.

In cases of head trauma, the ear should be evaluated in all of its components. A good understanding of otologic and skull base anatomy enables a thorough trauma assessment of this complex anatomic region. Auricular laceration, abrasion, avulsion, hematoma, frostbite, otitis externa, exostosis, tympanic membrane perforation, ossicular discontinuity, perilymphatic fistula, labyrinthine concussion, temporal bone fracture, facial nerve paresis, and sensorineural hearing loss are a few of the more common otologic injuries seen in active patients. Prevention of otologic trauma by wearing protective equipment during activity is the best way of maintaining the long-term health of the ear and audiovestibular function.

Nasal trauma is a common consequence of athletic competition. The nasal bones are the most commonly fractured facial bone and are particularly at risk during sports participation. Acute management of trauma to the nose includes thorough evaluation of all injuries and may require immediate management for repair of facial lacerations, epistaxis control, or septal hematoma drainage. Nasal fractures can often be addressed with closed reduction techniques; however, in the setting of complex nasal trauma, an open approach may be indicated. Using appropriate treatment techniques, posttraumatic nasal sequelae can be minimized; most patients report satisfactory long-term nasal form and function.

Sports account for 3% to 29% of facial injuries and 10% to 42% of facial fractures. Fractures of the facial skeleton most commonly occur owing to interpersonal violence or motor vehicle crashes. Facial fractures from sporting activities has clearly decreased over time owing to better preventive measures. However, this decreasing trend is offset by the emergence of more dangerous sports activities, or "pushing the envelope" of traditional sports activities. Fractures can occur from contact between athletes, and between athletes and their surroundings. Football, soccer, hockey, and baseball most frequently are involved in sports-related cases of facial bone fracture.

Oral and facial injuries are very common in sport, and can be very expensive to treat. Many of these injuries are preventable with proper precompetition assessment and suitable well-designed protection. Prompt sideline identification and management of orofacial injuries and appropriate follow-up are crucial to successful outcomes. There have been significant recent advances in both trauma management and mouth guard design and fabrication techniques. Athletes have a unique set of challenges—including collisions, finances, travel and training, dehydration, sport beverages, and high carbohydrate diets—that may compromise their oral health.

CLINICS IN SPORTS MEDICINE

RELATED INTEREST

Facial Plastic Surgery Clinics of North America, February 2017 (Vol. 25, Issue 1)
Facial Scar Management
David B. Hom, *Editor*
Available at: http://www.facialplastic.theclinics.com/

THE CLINICS ARE AVAILABLE ONLINE!
Access your subscription at:
www.theclinics.com

Foreword

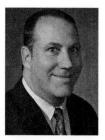

Mark D. Miller, MD
Consulting Editor

We developed this issue of *Clinics in Sports Medicine* to save face—literally! Dr
Michael Stuart, who has a wealth of experience in one of the most face-injury prone
sports there is, ice hockey, has put together this treatise on dealing with facial injuries
in sports. The issue begins with a discussion of epidemiology and prevention and then
presents an algorithmic approach to facial trauma. The issue then thoroughly and
comprehensively addresses specific facial injuries and their management. Thank
you, Dr Stuart, for taking on this difficult topic and providing guidance for those of
us taking care of patients with facial trauma!

Mark D. Miller, MD
Division of Sports Medicine
Department of Orthopaedic Surgery
University of Virginia
James Madison University
400 Ray C. Hunt Drive, Suite 330
Charlottesville, VA 22908-0159, USA

E-mail address:
mdm3p@virginia.edu

http://dx.doi.org/10.1016/j.csm.2017.01.002
0278-5919/17/© 2017 Published by Elsevier Inc.

sportsmed.theclinics.com

Preface

The Initial Evaluation and Treatment of Facial Injuries in Athletes

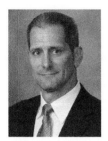

Michael J. Stuart, MD
Editor

*The **face** is the **most exposed body part** for athletes competing in many different sports.*

—*Michael J. Stuart, MD*

My greatest trepidation as a team physician who covers sporting events is the diagnosis and management of injuries to the cervical spine, brain, larynx, eye, and face. Sport-related facial injuries are common, representing approximately 40% of emergency department visits. The high-risk sports vary according to country, level of participation, and the use of facial protection. Fortunately, most of these injuries are mild, but some result in serious functional or cosmetic deficits. Facial trauma in sports may have significant consequences for both the individual and society.

We must all remember that prevention is the key. There is strong evidence to support the effectiveness of protective equipment and rule changes. For example, the use of full facial protection in the sport of ice hockey has virtually eliminated eye injuries. Missing legislation, noncompliance, and lack of enforcement can lead to significant risks to athletes in many sports, including permanent blindness.

Facial injuries in sports are caused by blunt, penetrating, or perforating mechanisms. The initial evaluation of an athlete with facial trauma begins with a focused assessment of the athlete's airway, breathing, and cervical spine. Resuscitative efforts are paramount, followed by a secondary evaluation for associated injuries to the brain, eye, and face.

Mouth guards are effective for decreasing the risk of oral trauma. Athletes should be encouraged to wear a custom-fit device for comfort, breathability, and optimal protection. Although there is no current scientific evidence to prove that mouth guards

Clin Sports Med 36 (2017) xi–xii
http://dx.doi.org/10.1016/j.csm.2017.01.001
0278-5919/17/© 2017 Published by Elsevier Inc.

prevent concussion or enhance performance, they should be worn with the goal of preventing dental injuries. In addition, a mouth guard may help stabilize the jaw and dissipate impact forces to the brain.

This special issue has been developed to provide a knowledge base for sports medicine providers so they can effectively recognize facial injuries, perform basic resuscitation, provide initial treatment, and refer to the appropriate specialist as indicated. Each of the expert authors offers a concise review along with practical tips that will help you promote safety, prevent catastrophic consequences, and ensure optimal results for your athletes.

Michael J. Stuart, MD
Department of Orthopedics
Division of Sports Medicine
Mayo Clinic
200 First Street, SW
Rochester, MN 55905, USA

E-mail address:
stuart.michael@mayo.edu

Epidemiology of Facial Injuries in Sport

Amanda M. Black, CAT(C), MSc[a,b,c], Paul H. Eliason, MSc[a,b,c], Declan A. Patton, PhD[a,b,c,d], Carolyn A. Emery, PT, PhD[a,b,c,e,*]

KEYWORDS

- Epidemiology • Facial injuries • Sport injuries • Eye injuries • Dental injuries
- Maxillofacial injuries

KEY POINTS

- Sport-related facial injuries can represent up to 41% of the injuries seen at emergency clinics.
- The top sports responsible for facial injuries vary depending on the country, and include baseball, basketball, floorball, soccer, tennis, rink bandy, and cycling.
- At present, understanding the burden of facial injuries in sport is challenging because studies are largely based on emergency room data and do not account for sport exposure time or participation rates.
- Future prospective studies that adjust for exposure and include standardized definitions of injuries are needed to better understand the risk and to evaluate the effectiveness of prevention programs.

INTRODUCTION

Participation in sport is associated with several health benefits.[1] However, there is also a risk of injury. Sport reportedly accounts for 4% to 41% of facial fractures,[2–11] 0.3% to 24% of eye injuries,[12–16] and 0.8% to 26% of dental injuries[17–21] evaluated at

Disclosure: The authors have no conflicts to disclose.
[a] Sport Injury Prevention Research Centre, Faculty of Kinesiology, University of Calgary, 2500 University Drive Northwest, Calgary, Alberta T2N 1N4, Canada; [b] Hotchkiss Brain Institute, Cumming School of Medicine, University of Calgary, Health Research Innovation Centre, Room 1A10, 3330 Hospital Drive Northwest, Calgary, Alberta T2N 4N1, Canada; [c] Alberta Children's Hospital Research Institute, Cumming School of Medicine, University of Calgary, Heritage Medical Research Building, Room 293, 3330 Hospital Drive Northwest, Calgary, Alberta T2N 4N1, Canada; [d] Australian Collaboration for Research into Injury in Sport and Its Prevention (ACRISP), Federation University, Lydiard Street South, Ballarat, Victoria 3350, Australia; [e] Departments of Pediatrics and Community Health Sciences, Cumming School of Medicine, University of Calgary, 2500 University Drive Northwest, Calgary, Alberta T2N 1N4, Canada
* Corresponding author. Sport Injury Prevention Research Centre, Faculty of Kinesiology, University of Calgary, 2500 University Drive Northwest, Calgary, Alberta T2N 1N4, Canada.
E-mail address: caemery@ucalgary.ca

Clin Sports Med 36 (2017) 237–255
http://dx.doi.org/10.1016/j.csm.2016.11.001
0278-5919/17/© 2016 Elsevier Inc. All rights reserved.

sportsmed.theclinics.com

emergency departments around the world. Estimating the risk of facial injuries in sport is complicated because there are many different types of facial injuries and different levels of reporting within each study. As shown in **Table 1** , the injury definition can vary widely between studies, across countries, and by age group. This article reviews the epidemiology of sport-related facial injuries as well as mechanisms of injury and facial injury risk factors.

MAXILLOFACIAL TRAUMA

The epidemiology of maxillofacial trauma has been examined in countries around the world. Studies of facial injuries in emergency departments in Italy, Chile, and Germany have identified soccer as having the highest frequency of sport-related facial fracture (41.6%–59.2%).[2,3,9] Specifically, the top sports resulting in maxillofacial and skull base fractures in Germany were soccer (59%), handball (8%), and inline-skating (7%).[9] However, in Italy, soccer (41.6%) and cycling (23.6%) were identified as the sports with the highest risk of facial trauma.[2] Maxillofacial injuries frequently involve the midface complex (67% overall, orbital floor fractures of the zygomatic bone [47%], nasal bone fractures [26%]) and the mandibular region (29%).[9] Mandible fractures most commonly occur at the condyle or just below the condyle. One study reported that 19 out of 42 sport-related mandible fractures treated at the maxillofacial clinic involved the condylar or sub-condylar region.[9] Compared with younger children, adolescents and young adults seem to be at greater risk for facial fractures.[6,7] Although men are reportedly more likely than women to visit the emergency department for a sport-related facial fracture,[3,7,10] these studies have not controlled for sport participation rates.

OCULAR INJURIES

The multiple types of eye injuries contribute to the complexity of assessing injury risk. A study examining sport-related eye injury in London, United Kingdom, reported that patients with sport-related eye injury most frequently present with traumatic uveitis, commotion retinae, traumatic hyphema, or corneal abrasion.[15] Another study from Helsinki, Finland, identified contusions as the most common injury.[12] Reports that include the incidence proportion (IP) of sport-related eye injuries are limited. The highest IP of sport-related eye injury in Helsinki, Finland, was found in rink bandy (IP, 0.05 per 100 athletes), floorball (IP, 0.047 per 100 athletes), tennis (IP, 0.047 per 100 athletes), baseball (IP, 0.04 per 100 athletes), and basketball (IP, 0.038 per 100 athletes).[12] In the United States, the top eye injury–producing sports were basketball (18%), baseball and softball (17%), and football (7%).[16] Soccer was responsible for the highest proportion of eye-related injuries presenting at emergency departments in Israel and London, United Kingdom.[14,15]

DENTAL INJURIES

Dental injury reports may include fractures, subluxations, avulsions, periodontal disease, abscess, pulpitis, and lacerations.[23] In a study examining the incidence and severity in 5 sports in the United States, basketball was identified as the sport with the highest dental injury rate.[24] Known risk factors for dental injuries include having a short upper lip and having an overjet greater than 3 to 4 mm.[17,23]

SPORT-SPECIFIC INJURY BURDEN

The IP, proportion of all injuries, risk factors, and common mechanisms of facial injury vary across sports. Sport characteristics, rules, and protective equipment can all

Table 1
Summary of studies published in the last 5 years that report on the proportion of facial injuries presenting at a hospital emergency room or clinic for sport-related injuries

Author	Country, Specific Location	Year	Specialized Clinic[a] (Yes/No)	Age (y)	Injuries Included	Sport-related Injuries/Total Injuries	Proportion Sport-related Injury (%)
Facial Fractures							
Arangio et al,[2] 2014	Italy, province of Latina, Lazio	2011–2012	No	All	Facial bone fractures (frontal bone, zygomatic complex, maxilla, nasal bone, orbit, mandible, panfascia), dentoalveolar trauma, and soft tissue injuries	10/79	13
Barrios et al,[3] 2013 (abstract)	Chile	2010–2012	NA	NA	Maxillofacial fractures (nasal, mandibular, orbital)	205/502 patients	40.9
Nardis et al,[4] 2013	Brazil, Sao Paulo	2008–2011	Yes	0–12	Facial fractures (nasal, mandible, zygomatic, maxilla, and dentoalveolar)	8/110	7.27
Kim et al,[5] 2012	Korea	2006–2010	No	<18	Facial fractures (nasal bone, maxilla, orbit, zygoma, mandible)	123/741	17
Paes et al,[6] 2012	Brazil, Lages, Santa Catarina	2003–2008	Yes	All	Facial fractures (mandibular bone, zygomatic complex, maxillary and nasal bone)	27/492	5.5
Muñante-Cárdenas et al,[7] 2011	Brazil, Sao Paulo	1999–2008	Yes	≤1	Facial fractures (mandible, maxillae, nasal bone, frontal bone, zygomatic bone, and nasal-orbital-ethmoid complex)	61/757	8.06

(continued on next page)

Table 1
(continued)

Author	Country, Specific Location	Year	Specialized Clinic[a] (Yes/No)	Age (y)	Injuries Included	Sport-related Injuries/Total Injuries	Proportion Sport-related Injury (%)
Chrcanovic et al,[8] 2010	Brazil, Belo Horizonte	2000–2002	Yes	≤18	Facial fractures (mandibular bone, zygomatic complex, maxillary and nasal bone)	35/464	7.54
Elhammali et al,[9] 2010	Germany, Bremen	2002–2007	Yes	All	Maxillofacial and skull base fractures (mandibular bone, zygomatic bone, orbital floor, nasal bone)	147/3596	4
Calderoni et al,[10] 2011	Brazil	2001–2008	Yes	4–82	Fracture of the orbitozygomatic complex	10/141	7
Muñante-Cárdenas et al,[22] 2010	Brazil, Sao Paulo	1999–2008	Yes	≤18	Mandibular fracture	6/108	5.36
Qing-Bin et al,[11] 2013	China	2000–2010	Yes	2–14	Maxillofacial injuries: soft tissue (gingiva, cheek, lip, chin, lateral face, palate/pharynx, nose, tongue/mouth floor, and forehead), fractures (mandible, maxilla, zygomatic bone, zygomatic arch, nasal, and orbital)	24/470	5.1

Eye Injuries						
Armstrong et al,[13] 2013	United States	2001–2007	No	0–17	Nonfatal injuries involving the eyeball (contusion/abrasion, foreign body, conjunctivitis, hemorrhage, burn, laceration/puncture, hematoma)	1285/15,326	9
Yulish et al,[14] 2013	Israel	2007–2011	Yes	6–58	Sport-related eye injuries (eyelid swelling, hematoma or lacerations, corneal erosions, conjunctival lacerations, hyphema, traumatic mydriasis, corneal perforation, macular edema)	323/16,991	2
Ong et al,[15] 2012	United Kingdom, London	2008 (May–July)	Yes	All	Sport-related eye injury (penetrating injury, choroidal rupture, retinal tear, retinal detachment, retinal hemorrhage, commotio retinae, vitreous hemorrhage, traumatic hyphema, traumatic uveitis, corneal abrasions, conjunctival laceration, orbital fracture, lid laceration, subconjunctival laceration)	48/16,999	0.28

(continued on next page)

Table 1
(continued)

Author	Country, Specific Location	Year	Specialized Clinic[a] (Yes/No)	Age (y)	Injuries Included	Sport-related Injuries/Total Injuries	Proportion Sport-related Injury (%)
Pollard et al,[16] 2012	United States	1990–2009	No	<18	Eye injuries (contusions/abrasions, conjunctivitis, foreign body, burns, punctures, lacerations, hemorrhage)	NA	24
Dental Injuries							
Stewart et al,[18] 2011	Ireland	2008	Yes	<18	Dental injury (crown fractures, lateral luxations, intrusions, avulsions, periodontal ligament)	39/168 teeth	23
Mohajerani et al,[19] 2011	Iran, Tehran	2006–2008	Yes	All	Midfacial fracture (Le Fort I, II, III; nasal bone; zygomatic; orbital floor; dentoalveolar; and mandibular)	2/243	0.80

| Diaz et al,[20] 2010 | Chile, Temuco | 2004–2007 | Yes | 1–15 | Dental injury (crown fractures; crown-root fracture; root fracture; alveolar bone fracture; periodontal tissue injuries; extrusive luxation; lateral luxation; intrusion, abrasions; lacerations of tongue, lips, cheek, or gingiva) | 31/359 | 8.60 |
| Hecova et al,[21] 2010 | Czech Republic | 1997–2002 | Yes | All | Dental injuries (crown-root fractures, concussion, subluxation, crown fractures, lateral luxation) | 100/384 | 26.0 |

Abbreviation: NA, information was not available in the article.
[a] Specialized clinic indicates that the emergency department specializes in seeing a particular type of injury.

affect injury risk. Information on the participation and risk of specific sports is provided here.

American Football

Facial injuries are uncommon in American football, accounting for less than 1% of all injuries.[25,26] The annual reported IP for eye injury in collegiate football is 0.1 injuries per 100 players.[27,28] Facial fractures do occur in American football; however, they comprise only 2% of all catastrophic injuries.[29]

Australian Football

Facial fractures comprise less than 2% of all injuries in Australian football,[30] with an associated incidence rate of less than 1.0 facial fractures per 1000 player-hours.[30,31]

Australian and Gaelic Football

Approximately 13% of all injuries in Australian football are to the face, resulting in an injury rate of 1 injury per 1000 player-hours.[32] Dental, nasal, and eye injuries are uncommon in Australian football and occur at a rates of less than 0.3 injuries per 1000 player-hours hours.[32] Facial fractures comprise 2% to 6% of all injuries in Australian football,[30,32] with an associated incidence of less than 1.0 facial fracture per 1000 player-hours.[30–32] Similarly, facial fractures are uncommon in Gaelic football, accounting for less than 1% of all injuries.[33]

Badminton

Badminton has been identified as a high-risk sport for eye injury.[34] However, similar to squash, because of limitations surrounding participation rates and prospective surveillance, understanding the risk of eye injury is challenging. For example, in a study of eye injuries presenting at emergency departments in Western Australia, badminton was listed as a sport producing eye injury but did not have a high enough incidence to report without combining with other sports.[35] In a study of patients presenting at an emergency eye clinic in Helsinki, Finland, 7 out of 149 (5%) sport-related cases were from badminton (IP, 0.014/100 athletes [0.26–0.77]).[12] Similarly, badminton involved 4.2% of the eye injuries seen at an emergency department in London, United Kingdom.[15] Information on the types of eye injuries sustained from badminton is limited. There is limited information on what types of eye injuries are sustained in badminton. One study reported that the most common type of eye injury is a contusion, accounting for all the injuries from badminton.[12]

Baseball and Softball

Although the rate of baseball-related injuries is one of the lowest among high school sports,[36] the face remains the most commonly injured body region presenting to US emergency departments despite the annual number of injuries presenting to the emergency department declining over time.[37,38] The most common injuries presented include lacerations (33%), contusions (30%), and fractures (27%), with the nose being the most common injury site.[37] The head and face (including mouth/teeth) accounted for approximately 16% of injuries of all high school baseball-related injuries, with a greater proportion of injuries to the head/face attributed to being hit by a batted ball (74%) than those not (9%).[36] Children (<8 years old) are more likely to be injured by the baseball bat, whereas older players are more likely to be injured by a baseball.[37] The incidence of eye injury is highest in children aged 5 to 14 years, with approximately one-third a result of being struck by a pitched ball.[39] Baseball had the third highest rate of rare injuries and conditions in high school athletes, with an eye and dental injury rate of 3.22/100,000 athlete exposures and 0.58/100,000 athlete exposures for neck and cervical injury.[40] Dental injury in intercollegiate players has an incidence rate of 0.5/100 athlete-seasons.[24] Fractures are typically caused by impact with the ball (68%) but can also be caused by collisions with another player (18%) and impact from a swung bat (13%).[41]

The number of softball injuries presenting annual to US emergency departments decreased from 1994 to 2005; however, there was an increase from 2005 to 2010.[42] The face was identified as the second most commonly injured body region, accounting for 19% of all injuries. Most facial injuries were lacerations (39%), soft tissue injuries (33%), or fractures/dislocations (22%).[42] Head and dental injuries accounted for 6% and 0.5% respectively, with most being head injuries (65%) as a result of concussions and closed head injuries. Being hit by the ball was the most common mechanism of injury, which accounted for 90% of face injuries, 76% of head injuries, and 95% of dental injuries.[42] Although the risk of injury has been claimed to be similar between softball and baseball,[39] softball seems to have a slightly lower rate than baseball of rare injuries and conditions in high school athletes. The rates of specific injury include eye injury (1.18 injuries per 100,000 athlete exposures), dental injury (0.39 injuries per 100,000 athlete exposures), and neck and cervical injury (0.39 injuries per 100,000 athlete exposures).[40] Most craniomaxillofacial fractures are caused by impact from the ball.[41,43]

Basketball

Basketball has been identified as a high-risk sport for both eye[5,34,40,44] and dental injuries.[24,40] In a survey of 388 basketball players from Brazil, 50% of the athletes had sustained orofacial injuries; 69.7% had sustained dental trauma; and 50.8% had sustained soft tissue injuries, including lip trauma, throughout their playing careers.[45] There was no relationship found between trauma and player position or facial type.[45] Facial fractures, lacerations, eye injuries, and dental injuries have been reported to make up between 1.1% and 2% of collegiate game injuries and between 1.2% and 4.0% of professional game injuries.[46–48] Injury rates have been reported to range from 0.1 to 0.8 facial lacerations per 1000 athlete exposures, 0.12 to 0.3 nasal fractures per 1000 athlete exposures, and 0.01 eye injuries per 1000 athlete exposures.[40,46–48] The most common type of eye injury in basketball is contusion[12] and the most common type of dental injury is a crown fracture.[24] Differences in the risk of dental injury rates between male and female basketball players may be caused by differences in enforcement regarding mouth guard use. For example, Cohenca and colleagues[24] reported a dental injury incidence of 10.6 injuries per 100 athlete-seasons for male basketball collegiate players between 1996 and 2006, and 5.0 per 100 athlete-seasons for female basketball players. One of the major reasons for the disparities between male and female basketball players in this study is that halfway through the collection period the women's basketball team introduced mandatory mouth guards, which resulted in a nonsignificant but noticeable 67% reduction in dental injuries (incidence rate ratio (IRR), 0.33; 95% confidence interval [CI], 0.03–2.33) after the women introduced mouth guards.[24] The most common mechanisms of orofacial injuries include contact with another player (91.8%), falling (5.67%), and a blow from the ball (5.15%).[45]

Boxing

Approximately 2% to 40% of all boxing injuries are sustained to the face in amateur boxing,[49,50] compared with professional boxing (66%–73%)[51–53] and female boxing

(78%–100%).[51,54] Facial injury rates reported in professional boxing range from 78 to 178 injuries per 1000 bouts[51–53] and in female boxing 23 to 49 injuries per 1000 bouts.[51,54] The most common types of facial injuries were lacerations and the most common location was the eye region (ie, eye, eyelid, and eyebrow).[50–54]

Floorball

According to the International Floorball Federation, floorball has been increasing in popularity over the last 30 years.[55] In 2015 there were approximately 310,000 licensed floorball players worldwide, with the highest participation rates in Sweden, Finland, and Czech Republic.[55] However, not all floorball players are licensed. It is estimated that around half a million people play floorball in Sweden at school, work, or through different associations.[56] According to prospective cohort studies, the most common injuries in floorball are joint sprains to the knee and ankle, with most studies reporting few or no facial injuries.[57,58] However, studies examining eye injuries specifically have identified floorball as a leading sport for eye injuries in Finland and Sweden.[12,59] In 2 studies examining patients presenting at an emergency eye clinic, 47 out of 149 (32%) and 167 out of 296 (56%) sport-related cases in Helsinki, Finland, and Jonkoping, Sweden, respectively were from floorball.[12,59] Leivo and colleagues[12] reported that the eye injury IP is 0.047 injuries per 100 athletes (95% CI, 0.034–0.062). The most common type of eye injury seen at eye clinics were contusions/edema (23%–94% of eye injuries),[12,59] hyphema (29% of eye injuries),[59] and dilated pupils (22% of eye injuries).[59] In floorball, the primary mechanisms of eye injuries include contact with the ball (69%–85%), contact with a stick (11%–22%), and contact with a body part (4%).[12,59] The focus on eye injuries is largely because, currently, eye protection is recommended but not required by the International Floorball Federation.[60]

Ice Hockey

Although rules regarding full/partial face protection and mouth guard use vary by league and country,[61,62] the incidence of head and face injuries in ice hockey has decreased because of the combination of mandatory use of full facial protection across many leagues and advancements in face shielding.[63–68] In men's International Ice Hockey Federation World Championship tournament play, head and face injuries were reported to represent 40% of all game-related injuries, with an injury rate of 5.7/1000 player-games.[69] Facial injuries alone comprised more than 70% of the head injuries, with an injury rate of 4.1/1000 player-games,[69] and the rate has been shown to be significantly higher among players wearing a half-shield visor (3.5/1000 athlete exposures) compared with those wearing full facial protection (1.41/1000 athlete exposures).[63] Most facial injuries are lacerations and are typically caused by high sticks.[63,69–71] The lip and eyebrow were the most frequent areas of laceration among those wearing a half-visor, and most were to the chin for those wearing full-face shields.[63,68] The rates of dental and eye injuries were 0.5/1000 player game-hours and 0.1/1000 player game-hours, respectively.[69] Fighting accounted for 12% of facial injuries in the East Coast Hockey League, with 5% occurring in players wearing a half-visor and 7% in those with no facial protection.[71]

Lacrosse

An estimated 22% of game injuries and 12% of practice injuries in lacrosse involve the head and neck.[72] Nasal fractures have been reported to make up 2.3% of injuries (IR, 0.1/1000 athlete exposures) in women's collegiate lacrosse.[72] Lacrosse has been placed in the high-risk category for eye injuries.[34] Eye contusions comprise 1.2% of game injuries (IR, 0.09/1000 athlete exposures and 1.3% of practice injuries (IR, 0.04/1000 athlete exposures) in women's collegiate lacrosse.[72] Head lacerations make up 1.3% of injuries in games (IR, 0.09/1000 athlete exposures).[72] The most common mechanism of injuries above the neck in lacrosse involved contact with the stick (56%).[72]

Mixed Martial Arts

The head is the most commonly injured anatomic region in mixed martial arts, accounting for approximately 67% to 78% of all injuries.[73] Blunt force to the head resulted in the highest proportion of match stoppages (28%) in a 10-year review, with periocular lacerations being the most common type of facial trauma.[74] The proportion of fighters that sustained documented ocular injuries was 10% and the proportion that sustained injuries of the face including suspected or probable fracture was 5% over a 5-year review.[75]

Rodeo

Research has shown that the head and neck is consistently one of the most commonly injured anatomic regions in high school and professional rodeo,[76–79] and accounts for between 10% and 29% of all injuries and up to 63% of injuries to the upper body.[80] The greatest injury frequency and injury incidence rates occur in the rough stock events, mainly bull riding and bareback riding.[76–78] The rate of head and neck injuries (including concussion) in professional bull riding is reportedly 8.7 injuries per 1000 rides (accounting for 27% of all injuries).[79] Another study reports a head and facial injury rate 15 injuries per 1000 rides.[81] However, it has been suggested that the rate may be even higher because of an underreporting of facial injuries.[82] Participation in rodeo, particularly bull riding, has the potential for catastrophic head injury, including permanent brain damage and impairment.[83] A documented series of 31 bull riders reported traumatic brain injury in Oklahoma over a 5-year period.[84] Mechanisms of injury differ depending on the rodeo event, with bull riders being more likely to sustain injuries to the head/face caused by colliding with the head or horns of the bull.[76,79] Other mechanisms of injury include being bucked off and hitting the ground, chute, or gate; getting stepped on; and being kicked.[77,79] Orofacial injuries in steer wrestling are usually caused by contact with the livestock's horn.[85,86]

Rugby League

Facial injury rates in youth rugby league[87] are reportedly 0.9 injuries per 1000 player-hours and, for adult[88] rugby league, 1.2 per 1000 player-hours, accounting for 9% to 14% of all injuries in amateur[89,90] and semiprofessional[91,92] competition. Specifically, injuries to the eyes and nose comprise 6.8% and 5.3% of all injuries, respectively.[93] Eye injuries have been found to comprise less than 4% of all injuries in junior rugby union players,[94] and nose injuries have been found to comprise 3% of all injuries in female rugby union players.[95] Mouth injuries comprised 9% and 2% of all rugby union injuries for adult male[93] and female[95] players respectively. In rugby league, facial fractures comprise approximately 4% of all injuries.[96] In Australia, the National Rugby League and National Youth Competition have slightly more than 10 facial fractures per season.[97,98]

Rugby union

Facial injuries comprise 16% of all injuries for adult male rugby union players[99] and 18% for female rugby union players.[100] Facial lacerations reportedly comprise 12%

and 3% of all injuries and occur at a rate of 0.44 injuries per 1000 athlete exposures for male collegiate rugby union players and 0.07 injuries per 1000 athlete exposures for female collegiate rugby union players, respectively.[101] Less than 5% of all male rugby union injuries[101] and less than 4% of all female rugby union injuries[100,101] involve the eyes. For youth rugby union players, facial injuries comprised 12% of all medical attention injuries, but less than 1% of all missed game injuries.[102] Approximately 4% of all injuries to female rugby players are mouth injuries and less than 1% of all injuries are dental injuries.[100] Facial fractures in rugby union comprise 12% of all catastrophic injuries[29]; however, less than 4% of all injuries in rugby union are facial fractures.[103–106]

Soccer

In soccer, facial injuries comprise 60% of all head injuries; however, most are of low severity.[107] Facial injuries comprise less than 6% and 3% for youth[108,109] and female[110,111] soccer players, respectively. Mouth injuries are uncommon and comprise approximately 2% of all injuries.[112] Facial fractures comprise 1% to 3% and 13% of all injuries[113,114] and all catastrophic injuries[29] respectively, with an associated injury rate of 0.4 facial fractures per 1000 player-hours.[113,114] In a study of patients presenting at an emergency clinic in Helsinki, Finland, 19 out of 149 sport-related cases were from soccer (IP, 0.019/100 athletes; 95% CI, 0.011–.029). The most common type of eye injury was a contusion (15 out of 19 injuries). The most common cause of eye injuries in soccer include being hit by the ball (83%) and by a body part (17%).[12]

Squash

Squash has been identified as having a moderate risk of both eye and dental injuries, primarily because of the rackets, close contact, and high velocity.[34,115] In studies of emergency departments, squash has been reported to be responsible for 0.7% of maxillofacial or skull base fractures in Germany,[9] and 10.4% of sport-related eye injuries seen in London, United Kingdom.[15] A survey of 600 amateur to professional squash players and coaches from Switzerland, Germany, and France reported a career IP for dental trauma of 4.5 injuries per 100 players.[115] The most common dental injury was a crown fracture (74% of all injuries), followed by an avulsion injury (22%).[115] Squash is often targeted as a sport for the prevention of eye injuries because the use of protective equipment is optional.[116] Prospective surveillance studies that account for participant exposure time are needed to better understand both the risk and the effectiveness of these interventions.

Taekwondo

In taekwondo, points are awarded for contact made to the head or body, with the highest points (4 points) awarded from a turning kick to the head.[117] Therefore, it is not surprising that an Olympic injury report identified taekwondo as having one of the highest injury IPs (12/100 athletes sustaining time-loss injuries and 39.1/100 athletes sustaining an injury requiring medical attention) at the London Summer Olympic Games.[118] Based on a questionnaire assessing the number of injuries over the last year in Australian taekwondo athletes, most injuries occurred during training rather than competition.[119] There are very few studies in taekwondo reporting on facial injuries specifically. A study in Turkey reported that 12 out of 50 (24%) taekwondo athletes self-reported experiencing some form of dental trauma.[120] The most common dental injury was a crown fracture.[120] Vidovic and colleagues[121] reviewed orofacial injuries in youth to adult (8–

28 years old) taekwondo athletes from Croatia. Out of the 484 participants, 300 (62%) had sustained an orofacial injury in the past. According to this report, men were more likely to sustain an injury participating in taekwondo than women.[121] Furthermore, senior (18–28 years old) taekwondo athletes were more likely to have sustained dental injuries.[121] However, this article did not control for exposure, and older athletes are more likely to have been competing for longer. One of the problems with estimates of injuries in taekwondo is that injuries may be underreported.[122] Poor recall, not believing the injury was important, and a desire to not disappoint their trainers have all been suggested as reasons contributing to these athletes' underestimation of injuries.[122]

Tennis

Very few studies have examined tennis injuries prospectively over the last decade. In the United States, no specific facial injuries were reported among collegiate athletes using the National Collegiate Athletic Association Injury Surveillance System.[123,124] However, tennis has been identified as having a moderate to high risk of eye injury by studies using emergency department databases.[34,125] For example, in a study of patients presenting at an emergency eye clinic in Helsinki, Finland, between 2011 and 2012, 15 out of 149 (10%) sport-related cases were from tennis (IP, 0.047/100 athletes; 95% CI, 0.026–0.077).[12] The rate of eye injuries presenting at US emergency departments between 2001 and 2009 was much lower (IP, 0.0077 per 100 athletes).[125] Tennis has been identified as being the sport responsible for between 2.5% and 10% of sport-related eye injuries presenting at the emergency department.[12,14,15] The most common types of eye injury in tennis are contusions[12] and hyphema.[35] The most common mechanism of eye injuries in tennis is the ball hitting the eye.[12,15,35]

SUMMARY

Facial injuries occur in many sports and can have catastrophic consequences for athletes. However, there are a limited number of prospective studies examining injury rates and risk factors for facial injury. Estimates of facial injury rates are complicated by a lack of, or inconsistent, reporting on specific types of injury. There is also a reliance on data from hospitals that specialize in a specific type of injury, which may overestimate the incidence of that specific injury. Using hospital-based data, the risk caused by sport varies by country, depending on the popularity of sports in that region. Many studies report only time-loss injuries and thus milder injuries, including lacerations and contusions, may not be included. In addition, there are minimal data evaluating sport-specific risk factors. Prospective injury surveillance studies with consistent injury definitions examining risk factors and controlling for exposure to risk (participation exposures or hours) are needed to better understand the burden of facial injuries in sport and the effectiveness of facial injury prevention efforts.

REFERENCES

1. Zullig KJ, White RJ. Physical activity, life satisfaction, and self-rated health of middle school students. Appl Res Qual Life 2010;6(3):277–89.
2. Arangio P, Vellone V, Torre U, et al. Maxillofacial fractures in the province of Latina, Lazio, Italy: review of 400 injuries and 83 cases. J Craniomaxillofac Surg 2014;42(5):583–7.
3. Barrios J, Teuber C, Cosmelli R. Prevalence of sports-related maxillofacial fractures, at Clinica Alemana Santiago, Chile. Int J Oral Maxillofac Surg 2013; 42(10):1220.

4. Nardis A, da C, Costa SAP, et al. Patterns of paediatric facial fractures in a hospital of São Paulo, Brazil: a retrospective study of 3 years. J Craniomaxillofac Surg 2013;41(3):226-9.
5. Kim SH, Lee SH, Cho PD. Analysis of 809 facial bone fractures in a pediatric and adolescent population. Arch Plast Surg 2012;39(6):606.
6. Paes JV, de Sá Paes FL, Valiati R, et al. Retrospective study of prevalence of face fractures in southern Brazil. Indian J Dent Res 2012;23(1):80-6.
7. Muñante-Cárdenas JL, Olate S, Asprino L, et al. Pattern and treatment of facial trauma in pediatric and adolescent patients. J Craniofac Surg 2011;22(4):1251-5.
8. Chrcanovic BR, Abreu MHNG, Freire-Maia B, et al. Facial fractures in children and adolescents: a retrospective study of 3 years in a hospital in Belo Horizonte, Brazil. Dent Traumatol 2010;26(3):262-70.
9. Elhammali N, Bremerich A, Rustemeyer J. Demographical and clinical aspects of sports-related maxillofacial and skull base fractures in hospitalized patients. Int J Oral Maxillofac Surg 2010;39(9):857-62.
10. Calderoni DR, Guidi Mde C, Kharmandayan P, et al. Seven-year institutional experience in the surgical treatment of orbito-zygomatic fractures. J Craniomaxillofac Surg 2011;39(8):593-9.
11. Qing-Bin Z, Zhao-Qiang Z, Dan C, et al. Epidemiology of maxillofacial injury in children under 15 years of age in southern China. Oral Surg Oral Med Oral Pathol Oral Radiol 2013;115(4):436-41.
12. Leivo T, Haavisto A-K, Sahraravand A. Sports-related eye injuries: the current picture. Acta Ophthalmol 2015;93(3):224-31.
13. Armstrong GW, Kim JG, Linakis JG, et al. Pediatric eye injuries presenting to United States emergency departments: 2001-2007. Graefes Arch Clin Exp Ophthalmol 2013;251(3):629-36.
14. Yulish M, Reshef N, Lerner A, et al. Sport-related eye injury in northern Israel. Isr Med Assoc J 2013;15(12):763-5.
15. Ong HS, Barsam A, Morris OC, et al. A survey of ocular sports trauma and the role of eye protection. Cont Lens Anterior Eye 2012;35(6):285-7.
16. Pollard KA, Xiang H, Smith GA. Pediatric eye injuries treated in us emergency departments, 1990-2009. Clin Pediatr 2012;51(4):374-81.
17. Ain TS, Lingesha RT, Sultan S, et al. Prevalence of traumatic dental injuries to anterior teeth of 12-year-old school children in Kashmir, India. Arch Trauma Res 2016;5(1):e24596.
18. Stewart C, Kinirons M, Delaney P. Clinical audit of children with permanent tooth injuries treated at a dental hospital in Ireland. Eur Arch Paediatr Dent 2011; 12(1):41-5.
19. Mohajerani SH, Asghari S. Pattern of mid-facial fractures in Tehran, Iran. Dent Traumatol 2011;27(2):131-4.
20. Díaz JA, Bustos L, Brandt AC, et al. Dental injuries among children and adolescents aged 1-15 years attending to public hospital in Temuco, Chile. Dent Traumatol 2010;26(3):254-61.
21. Hecova H, Tzigkounakis V, Merglova V, et al. A retrospective study of 889 injured permanent teeth. Dent Traumatol 2010;26(6):466-75.
22. Muñante-Cárdenas JL, Asprino L, De Moraes M, et al. Mandibular fractures in a group of Brazilian subjects under 18 years of age: a epidemiological analysis. Int J Pediatr Otorhinolaryngol 2010;74(11):1276-80.
23. Inouye J, McGrew C. Dental problems in athletes. Curr Sports Med Rep 2015; 14(1):27-33.

24. Cohenca N, Roges RA, Roges R. The incidence and severity of dental trauma in intercollegiate athletes. J Am Dent Assoc 2007;138(8):1121–6.
25. Badgeley MA, McIlvain NM, Yard EE, et al. Epidemiology of 10,000 high school football injuries: patterns of injury by position played. J Phys Act Health 2013; 10(2):160–9.
26. Willigenburg NW, Borchers JR, Quincy R, et al. Comparison of injuries in American collegiate football and club rugby: a prospective cohort study. Am J Sports Med 2016;44(3):753–60.
27. Dick R, Agel J, Marshall SW. National Collegiate Athletic Association injury surveillance system commentaries: introduction and methods. J Athl Train 2007; 42(2):173–82.
28. Olson D, Sikka R, Pulling T, et al. Eye injuries in sport. In: Madden C, Putukian M, Young C, et al, editors. Netter's sports medicine. Section VII: injury prevention, diagnosis, and treatment. 1st edition. Philadelphia: Saunders; 2010. p. 332–9.
29. Saleh F, Jalal A. Section 7: field sports. In: Tator CH, editor. Catastrophic injuries in sports and recreation: causes and prevention - a Canadian study. Toronto: University of Toronto Press; 2008. p. 457–82.
30. Savage J, Winter M, Orchard J, et al. Incidence of facial fractures in the Australian Football League. ANZ J Surg 2012;82(10):724–8. http://dx.doi.org/10.1111/j.1445-2197.2012.06181.x.
31. Orchard J, Seward H. Epidemiology of injuries in the Australian Football League, seasons 1997-2000. Br J Sports Med 2002;36(1):39–44.
32. Braham R, Finch C, McCrory P. The incidence of head/neck/orofacial injuries in non-elite Australian football. J Sci Med Sport 2004;7(4):451–3.
33. Blake C, John M, Conor G, et al. Injury to the head region in elite male Gaelic football and hurling: 2007-2012. Br J Sports Med 2014;48(7):569.
34. Dain SJ. Sports eyewear protective standards. Clin Exp Optom 2016;99(1): 4–23.
35. Hoskin AK, Yardley A-ME, Hanman K, et al. Sports-related eye and adnexal injuries in the Western Australian paediatric population. Acta Ophthalmol 2016; 94(6):e407–10.
36. Collins CL, Comstock RD. Epidemiological features of high school baseball injuries in the United States, 2005-2007. Pediatrics 2008;121(6):1181–7.
37. Carniol ET, Shaigany K, Svider PF, et al. "Beaned": a 5-year analysis of baseball-related injuries of the face. Otolaryngol Head Neck Surg 2015;153(6):957–61.
38. Lawson BR, Comstock RD, Smith GA. Baseball-related injuries to children treated in hospital emergency departments in the United States, 1994-2006. Pediatrics 2009;123(6):e1028–34.
39. Committee on Sports Medicine and Fitness. American Academy of Pediatrics. Risk of injury from baseball and softball in children. Pediatrics 2001;107:782.
40. Huffman EA, Yard EE, Fields SK, et al. Epidemiology of rare injuries and conditions among United States high school athletes during the 2005-2006 and 2006-2007 school years. J Athl Train 2008;43(6):624–30.
41. Bak MJ, Doerr TD. Craniomaxillofacial fractures during recreational baseball and softball. J Oral Maxillofac Surg 2004;62(10):1209–12.
42. Birchak JC, Rochette LM, Smith GA. Softball injuries treated in US EDs, 1994 to 2010. Am J Emerg Med 2013;31(6):900–5.
43. Yamamoto K, Murakami K, Sugiura T, et al. Maxillofacial fractures sustained during baseball and softball. Dent Traumatol 2009;25(2):194–7.
44. Pieper P. Epidemiology and prevention of sports-related eye injuries. J Emerg Nurs 2010;36(4):359–61.

45. Frontera RR, Zanin L, Ambrosano GMB, et al. Orofacial trauma in Brazilian basketball players and level of information concerning trauma and mouthguards. Dent Traumatol 2011;27(3):208–16.

46. Deitch JR, Starkey C, Walters SL, et al. Injury risk in professional basketball players: a comparison of Women's National Basketball Association and National Basketball Association athletes. Am J Sports Med 2006;34(7):1077–83.

47. Agel J, Olson DE, Dick R, et al. Descriptive epidemiology of collegiate women's basketball injuries: National Collegiate Athletic Association Injury Surveillance System, 1988-1989 through 2003-2004. J Athl Train 2007;42(2):202–10.

48. Dick R, Hertel J, Agel J, et al. Descriptive epidemiology of collegiate men's basketball injuries: National Collegiate Athletic Association Injury Surveillance System, 1988-1989 through 2003-2004. J Athl Train 2007;42(2):194–201.

49. Loosemore M, Lightfoot J, Palmer-Green D, et al. Boxing injury epidemiology in the Great Britain team: a 5-year surveillance study of medically diagnosed injury incidence and outcome. Br J Sports Med 2015;49(17):1100–7.

50. Siewe J, Rudat J, Zarghooni K, et al. Injuries in competitive boxing. A prospective study. Int J Sports Med 2015;36(3):249–53.

51. Bledsoe GH, Li G, Levy F. Injury risk in professional boxing. South Med J 2005; 98(10):994–8.

52. Zazryn TR, McCrory PR, Cameron PA. Injury rates and risk factors in competitive professional boxing. Clin J Sport Med 2009;19(1):20–5.

53. Zazryn TR, Finch CF, McCrory P. A 16 year study of injuries to professional boxers in the state of Victoria, Australia. Br J Sports Med 2003;37(4):321–4.

54. Bianco M, Pannozzo A, Fabbricatore C, et al. Medical survey of female boxing in Italy in 2002-2003. Br J Sports Med 2005;39(8):532–6.

55. International Floorball Federation. Number of licensed players 2015 – 09.03.2016. 2016. Available at: http://www.floorball.org/news.asp?tyyppi=kohdennettu&alue=204&id_tiedote=4836. Accessed May 25, 2016.

56. Tervo T, Nordström A. Science of floorball: a systematic review. Open Access J Sport Med 2014;5:249–55.

57. Tranaeus U, Götesson E, Werner S. Injury profile in Swedish elite floorball: a prospective cohort study of 12 teams. Sports Health 2016;8(3):224–9.

58. Pasanen K, Parkkari J, Kannus P, et al. Injury risk in female floorball: a prospective one-season follow-up. Scand J Med Sci Sports 2008;18(1):49–54.

59. Bro T, Ghosh F. Floorball-related eye injuries: the impact of protective eyewear. Scand J Med Sci Sports 2016. [Epub ahead of print].

60. International Floorball Federation. CE-marking of protective eyewear used in the game of floorball. 2007. Available at: http://floorball.sp.se/en/protective_eyewear/Sidor/default.aspx. Accessed May 27, 2016.

61. USA Hockey. Official rules of ice hockey. 2013. Available at: http://assets.ngin.com/attachments/document/0042/4244/2013-17_USAH_Rulebook.pdf. Accessed May 1, 2016.

62. Hockey Canada. Referee's case book/rule combination 2014-2015. 2014. Available at: http://www.hockeycanada.ca/en-ca/Hockey-Programs/Officiating/Essentials/Downloads.aspx. Accessed July 16, 2015.

63. Benson BW. Head and neck injuries among ice hockey players wearing full face shields vs half face shields. JAMA 1999;282(24):2328.

64. Pashby T. Eye injuries in Canadian amateur hockey still a concern. Can J Ophthalmol 1987;22(6):293–5.

65. Pashby TJ. Eye injuries in Canadian amateur hockey. Am J Sports Med 1979; 7(4):254–7.

66. Biasca N, Simmen HP, Trentz O. Head injuries in ice hockey exemplified by the National Hockey League "Hockey Canada" and European teams. Unfallchirurg 1993;96(5):259–64 [in German].
67. Lawrence LA, Svider PF, Raza SN, et al. Hockey-related facial injuries: a population-based analysis. Laryngoscope 2015;125(3):589–93.
68. LaPrade RF, Burnett QM, Zarzour R, et al. The effect of the mandatory use of face masks on facial lacerations and head and neck injuries in ice hockey. A prospective study. Am J Sports Med 1995;23(6):773–5.
69. Tuominen M, Stuart MJ, Aubry M, et al. Injuries in men's international ice hockey: a 7-year study of the International Ice Hockey Federation Adult World Championship Tournaments and Olympic Winter Games. Br J Sports Med 2015;49(1):30–6.
70. Stuart MJ, Smith A. Injuries in junior A ice hockey: a three-year prospective study. Am J Sports Med 1995;23(4):458–61.
71. Bunn JW. Changing the face of hockey: a study of the half-visor's ability to reduce the severity of facial injuries of the upper-half of the face among east coast hockey league players. Phys Sportsmed 2008;36(1):76–86.
72. Dick R, Lincoln AE, Agel J, et al. Descriptive epidemiology of collegiate women's lacrosse injuries: National Collegiate Athletic Association Injury Surveillance System, 1988-1989 through 2003-2004. J Athl Train 2007;42(2):262–9.
73. Lystad RP, Gregory K, Wilson J. The epidemiology of injuries in mixed martial arts: a systematic review and meta-analysis. Orthop J Sports Med 2014;2(1). 2325967113518492.
74. Buse GJ. No holds barred sport fighting: a 10 year review of mixed martial arts competition. Br J Sports Med 2006;40(2):169–72.
75. Ngai KM, Levy F, Hsu EB. Injury trends in sanctioned mixed martial arts competition: a 5-year review from 2002 to 2007. Br J Sports Med 2008;42(8):686–9.
76. Mobile Sport Medicine System. Mobile sport medicine system 25 year injury study. 2005. Available at: http://www.msmsinc.com/injurystats.html. Accessed May 1, 2016.
77. Sinclair AJ, Smidt C. Analysis of 10 years of injury in high school rodeo. Clin J Sport Med 2009;19(5):383–7.
78. Butterwick DJ, Hagel B, Nelson DS, et al. Epidemiologic analysis of injury in five years of Canadian professional rodeo. Am J Sports Med 2002;30(2):193–8.
79. Butterwick DJ, Meeuwisse WH. Bull riding injuries in professional rodeo: data for prevention and care. Phys Sportsmed 2003;31(6):37–41.
80. Meyers MC, Laurent CM. The rodeo athlete: injuries - Part II. Sports Med 2010; 40(10):817–39.
81. Brandenburg MA, Archer P. Survey analysis to assess the effectiveness of the bull tough helmet in preventing head injuries in bull riders: a pilot study. Clin J Sport Med 2002;12(6):360–6.
82. Larrison WI, Hersh PS, Kunzweiler T, et al. Sports-related ocular trauma. Ophthalmology 1990;97(10):1265–9.
83. Andrews DM, Brett K, Bugg BH, et al. Agreement statement from the 1st International Rodeo Research and Clinical Care Conference. Clin J Sport Med 2005; 15(3):192–5.
84. Brandenburg MA, Schmidt A, Mallonee S. Bull-riding Injuries. Ann Emerg Med 1998;32(1):118.
85. Meyers MC, Laurent CM. The rodeo athlete: injuries - Part I. Sports Med 2010; 40(10):817–39.
86. Meyers MC, Elledge JR, Sterling JC, et al. Injuries in intercollegiate rodeo athletes. Am J Sports Med 1990;18(1):87–91.

87. Gabbett TJ. Incidence of injury in junior rugby league players over four competitive seasons. J Sci Med Sport 2008;11(3):323–8.
88. Gabbett TJ, Domrow N. Risk factors for injury in subelite rugby league players. Am J Sports Med 2005;33(3):428–34.
89. Gabbett TJ. Incidence, site, and nature of injuries in amateur rugby league over three consecutive seasons. Br J Sports Med 2000;34(2):98–103.
90. Gabbett TJ. Severity and cost of injuries in amateur rugby league: a case study. J Sports Sci 2001;19(5):341–7.
91. Gabbett TJ. Incidence of injury in semi-professional rugby league players. Br J Sports Med 2003;37(1):36–43 [discussion: 43–4].
92. Gabbett TJ. Influence of training and match intensity on injuries in rugby league. J Sports Sci 2004;22(5):409–17.
93. King D, Gabbett TJ. Amateur rugby league match injuries in New Zealand. New Zeal J Sport Med 2009;36(1):16–21.
94. King DA. Incidence of injuries in the 2005 New Zealand national junior rugby league competition. New Zeal Jounal Sport Med 2006;34(1):21–7.
95. King DA, Gabbett TJ. Injuries in a national women's rugby league tournament: an initial investigation. NZ J Sport Med 2007;34(2):2–5.
96. King D, Hume P, Gianotti S, et al. A retrospective review over 1999 to 2007 of head, shoulder and knee soft tissue and fracture dislocation injuries and associated costs for rugby league in New Zealand. Int J Sports Med 2011;32(4):287–91.
97. O'Connor D. NRL injury report 2010. Sports Health 2011;29(1):17–25.
98. O'Connor D. NRL injury report 2011. Sports Health 2012;30(1):12–22.
99. Schneiders AG, Takemura M, Wassinger CA. A prospective epidemiological study of injuries to New Zealand premier club rugby union players. Phys Ther Sport 2009;10(3):85–90.
100. Comstock RD. Patterns of injury among female rugby players. San Diego (CA): University of California; 2002.
101. Peck KY, Johnston DA, Owens BD, et al. The incidence of injury among male and female intercollegiate rugby players. Sports Health 2013;5(4):327–33.
102. McIntosh AS, McCrory P, Finch CF, et al. Head, face and neck injury in youth rugby: incidence and risk factors. Br J Sports Med 2010;44(3):188–93.
103. Bottini E, Poggi EJ, Luzuriaga F, et al. Incidence and nature of the most common rugby injuries sustained in Argentina (1991-1997). Br J Sports Med 2000;34(2):94–7.
104. Brooks JHM, Fuller CW, Kemp SPT, et al. A prospective study of injuries and training amongst the England 2003 Rugby World Cup squad. Br J Sports Med 2005;39(5):288–93.
105. Brooks JHM, Fuller CW, Kemp SPT, et al. Epidemiology of injuries in English professional rugby union: part 1 match injuries. Br J Sports Med 2005;39(10):757–66.
106. Willigenburg NW, Geissler KE, Benjamin D, et al. Injuries in American Collegiate Club Rugby: a prospective study. Ann Sports Med Res 2014;(1):1005.
107. Correa MB, Knabach CB, Collares K, et al. Video analysis of craniofacial soccer incidents: a prospective study. J Sci Med Sport 2012;15(1):14–8.
108. Brito J, Malina RM, Seabra A, et al. Injuries in Portuguese youth soccer players during training and match play. J Athl Train 2012;47(2):191–7.
109. Pangrazio O, Forriol F. Epidemiology of injuries sustained by players during the 16th under-17 South American Soccer Championship. Rev Esp Cir Ortop Traumatol 2016;60(3):192–9.

110. Meyers MC. Incidence, mechanisms, and severity of match-related collegiate women's soccer injuries on FieldTurf and natural grass surfaces: a 5-year prospective study. Am J Sports Med 2013;41(10):2409–20.
111. Tegnander A, Olsen OE, Moholdt TT, et al. Injuries in Norwegian female elite soccer: a prospective one-season cohort study. Knee Surg Sports Traumatol Arthrosc 2008;16(2):194–8.
112. Hassabi M, Mohammad-Javad Mortazavi S, Giti M-R, et al. Injury profile of a professional soccer team in the Premier League of Iran. Asian J Sports Med 2010; 1(4):201–8.
113. Andersen TE, Tenga A, Engebretsen L, et al. Video analysis of injuries and incidents in Norwegian professional football. Br J Sports Med 2004;38(5):626–31.
114. Andersen TE, Arnason A, Engebretsen L, et al. Mechanisms of head injuries in elite football. Br J Sports Med 2004;38(6):690–6.
115. Persic R, Pohl Y, Filippi A. Dental squash injuries - a survey among players and coaches in Switzerland, Germany and France. Dent Traumatol 2006;22(5): 231–6.
116. Eime R, Finch C, Wolfe R, et al. The effectiveness of a squash eyewear promotion strategy. Br J Sports Med 2005;39(9):681–5.
117. World Taekwondo Federation. World Taekwondo Federation competition rules & interpretation. 2015. Available at: http://www.worldtaekwondofederation.net/wp-content/uploads/2015/11/WTF_Competition_Rules__Interpretation_May_11_2015.pdf. Accessed May 18, 2016.
118. Engebretsen L, Steffen K, Alonso JM, et al. Sports injuries and illnesses during the London Summer Olympic Games 2012. Br J Sports Med 2013;44(11): 772–80.
119. Lystad R, Graham P, Poulos R. Epidemiology of training injuries in amateur taekwondo athletes: a retrospective cohort study. Biol Sport 2015;32(3):213–8.
120. Keçeci AD, Eroglu E, Baydar ML. Dental trauma incidence and mouthguard use in elite athletes in Turkey. Dent Traumatol 2005;21(2):76–9.
121. Vidovic D, Bursac D, Skrinjaric T, et al. Prevalence and prevention of dental injuries in young taekwondo athletes in Croatia. Eur J Paediatr Dent 2015;16(2): 107–10.
122. Kazemi M, Shearer H, Choung YS. Pre-competition habits and injuries in Taekwondo athletes. BMC Musculoskelet Disord 2005;6:26.
123. Youn J, Sallis RE, Smith G, et al. Ocular injury rates in college sports. Med Sci Sports Exerc 2008;40(3):428–32.
124. Lynall RC, Kerr ZY, Djoko A, et al. Epidemiology of National Collegiate Athletic Association men's and women's tennis injuries, 2009/2010–2014/2015. Br J Sports Med 2015;50(7):1–6.
125. Kim T, Nunes AP, Mello MJ, et al. Incidence of sports-related eye injuries in the United States: 2001-2009. Graefes Arch Clin Exp Ophthalmol 2011;249(11): 1743–4.

Prevention of Sport-related Facial Injuries

Amanda M. Black, CAT(C), MSc[a,b,c], Declan A. Patton, PhD[a,b,c,d],
Paul H. Eliason, MSc[a,b,c], Carolyn A. Emery, PT, PhD[a,b,c,e],*

KEYWORDS

- Epidemiology • Prevention • Facial injuries • Sport injuries • Eye injuries
- Dental injuries • Maxillofacial injuries

KEY POINTS

- Strong evidence surrounding the effectiveness of protective equipment and rule changes is limited.
- Rule changes mandating mouth guards and eye protection have been effective at reducing the risk of oral and eye trauma.
- Protective standards can assist with ensuring the equipment purchased is capable of withstanding the forces of the sport, but the difference between equipment that meets the standard and equipment that does not meet the standard has not been evaluated using prospective studies.
- Mouth guard use, regardless of type, is associated with a reduction in oral trauma but custom-fitted mouth guards may increase comfort and breathability, and may offer superior protection.

INTRODUCTION

Sport-related facial injuries represent more than 41% of the injuries seen at emergency clinics.[1-20] Such injuries often result in surgical procedures that lead to extended periods of time away from sport and can be potentially career ending.

Disclosure: The authors have no conflicts to disclose.
[a] Sport Injury Prevention Research Centre, Faculty of Kinesiology, University of Calgary, 2500 University Drive Northwest, Calgary, Alberta T2N 1N4, Canada; [b] Hotchkiss Brain Institute, Cumming School of Medicine, University of Calgary, Health Research Innovation Centre, Room 1A10, 3330 Hospital Drive Northwest, Calgary, Alberta T2N 4N1, Canada; [c] Alberta Children's Hospital Research Institute, Cumming School of Medicine, University of Calgary, Heritage Medical Research Building, Room 293, 3330 Hospital Drive Northwest, Calgary, Alberta T2N 4N1, Canada; [d] Australian Collaboration for Research into Injury in Sport and Its Prevention (ACRISP), Federation University, Lydiard Street South, Ballarat, Victoria 3350, Australia; [e] Departments of Pediatrics and Community Health Sciences, Cumming School of Medicine, University of Calgary, 2500 University Drive Northwest, Calgary, Alberta T2N 1N4, Canada
* Corresponding author. Sport Injury Prevention Research Centre, Faculty of Kinesiology, University of Calgary, 2500 University Drive Northwest, Calgary, Alberta T2N 1N4, Canada.
E-mail address: caemery@ucalgary.ca

Primary prevention strategies are essential for continued participation in sport and the general health of athletes. This article evaluates some of the strategies used for the prevention of sport-related eye injuries, oral injuries, and overall facial injuries, as well as providing sport-specific considerations in preventive measures.

EYE PROTECTION

Understanding the full effect of wearing eye protection is difficult because of the lack of accurate and consistent injury surveillance with consideration of exposure to risk (ie, participation exposures or hours).[21] Features of sports that may place athletes at higher risk of eye injury include balls, bats, and sticks that come into close range or contact.[21] Strategies to reduce eye injuries include rule changes and eye protection equipment.

In 2004, the American Academy of Pediatrics and the American Academy of Ophthalmology recommended protective eyewear for all youth participating in baseball/softball, basketball, bicycling, boxing, fencing, field hockey, football, full-contact martial arts, ice hockey, lacrosse, paintball, racquet sports, soccer, street hockey, track and field, water polo/swimming, and wrestling.[22] However, very few of those sports have mandatory eye protection and it is often up to the players to regulate their use.

Several standards for sport eye protection exist in Australia and New Zealand,[23] Canada,[24] the United Kingdom,[25] and the United States.[26] Such standards are primarily intended for racquet sports; however, some identify other sports for which they are appropriate (eg, lacrosse, field hockey, basketball, baseball, and soccer).[26,27] In the United States, field hockey[28] and women' lacrosse[29] have additional standards for eye protection. Eye protection is often made with polycarbonate plastic at least 3 mm thick, which is both durable and impact resistant.[30] Prescription glasses and contact lenses do not adequately prevent eye injuries, and may introduce additional injury risk.[30,31]

Mandatory eye protection has been examined in floorball, lacrosse, and field hockey. This rule enforcement has been found to be effective in reducing injury risk by 69% to 84% and has led to a dramatic reduction in eye injuries seen in the emergency department (**Table 1**).[32,33]

Although it is clear that protective eyewear is effective at preventing eye injuries, participants may choose not to wear it for several reasons. These reasons may include lack of interest, discomfort, disruption of their sight, wearing prescription glasses, not believing there is a risk, or simply a preference to not wear them.[34–36] Educational efforts have shown some effectiveness at changing protective eyewear behavior, but such efforts have not been linked to injury reduction.[37]

ORAL PROTECTION

The goal of a mouth guard is to dissipate the force between the upper and lower teeth and act as a shock absorber,[30,38] which can help protect the lips and tissue inside the mouth from laceration as well as the teeth and the jaw from dislocation.[38] There are 3 types of mouth guards: custom-fabricated guards made by dental professionals using a model of the patient's teeth and vacuum-forming or heat-pressure lamination; form-fitted, boil-and-bite guards made by the athlete biting the mouth guard; stock guards, bought directly over the counter for immediate wear.[38]

The American Dental Association recommends that mouth guards be worn in any sport that poses a risk to the mouth, including acrobatics, basketball, boxing, equestrian events, extreme sports, field hockey, football, gymnastics, handball, ice hockey,

Table 1
Summary of studies examining the effectiveness of eye protection

Author and Year	Sport/Study Design/ Years Studied/Country	Outcome (Injury Types Included)	Participants (Level, Sex, Age, Sample Size)	Intervention and Control Description	Reported IR (per 1000 h) or IP (per 100 Players)	Effect Estimates Reported or Calculated Based on Data Provided
Kriz et al,[32] 2015	Field hockey/Historical cohort/2009–2013/ United States	Eye and orbital injuries Head/face injuries	High school Female CG: N = 156 IG: N = 117	NFHS initiated MPE in 2011 CG: No MPE IG: MPE	Eye injury IG: IR = 0.025 per 1000 AE CG: IR = 0.080 per 1000 AE Head/face IG: IR = 0.252 per 1000 AE CG: IR = 0.323 per 1000 AE	Eye injuries OR[a] = 0.31 (0.14–0.68) Head/face OR[a] = 0.78 (0.58–1.05)
Lincoln et al,[33] 2012	Lacrosse/Historical cohort/2000–2009	Eye injuries: globe, eyelid, eyebrow, eye orbit Head/face injuries: nose, mouth, teeth, tongue, face, forehead, cheek, chin, jaw, head (nonconcussion)	High school Female	US lacrosse mandated protective eyewear CG: no MPE IG: MPE	Eye injuries IG MPE: 0.016 per 1000 AE CG no MPE: 0.10 per 1000 AE	Eye injuries RR = 0.16 (0.06–0.42) Head/face injuries RR = 0.44 (0.26–0.76)

Abbreviations: AE, athlete-exposures; CG, control group; IG, intervention group or those exposed to the prevention strategy; IP, incidence proportion; IR, incidence rate; IRR, incidence rate ratio; MPE, mandatory protective eyewear; n, number of players; N, number of teams; NFHS, National Federation of State High School Associations; OR, odds ratio (95% confidence interval [CI] where available); RR, risk ratio.
[a] OR was inversed.

lacrosse, martial arts, racquetball, rugby, skiing, soccer, softball, squash, volleyball, water polo, weightlifting, and wrestling.[39] However, mandatory mouth guard policies occur primarily at the international level and the amateur level has little enforcement.[30,40] For example, despite mandated mouth guards by the National Collegiate Athletic Association (NCAA) in ice hockey in 1998, it was estimated that only 63% of athletes wore mouth guards during games.[40]

Several standards exist for mouth guards in the United States,[41–43] but standards in other regions are only in the preliminary stage[44] or have been withdrawn.[45,46] Furthermore, mouth guards do not need to meet standards to be sold. In a study examining commercially available mouth guard material (eg, Essix Resin, Erkoflex, Proform-regular, Proform-laminate, and Polyshok), none of the materials tested met the requirements of the American National Standards Institute (ANSI) or Standards Australia International (SAI) for impact attenuation.[47] It is also important to note that mouth guards may need to be replaced regularly to ensure substantial protection. Del Rossi and colleagues[48] examined changes to mouth guards in high school football players throughout a season and found that thickness decreased by 16% in the incisor/canine region and 23% in the molar region after 16 weeks. Specific recommendations informing when a mouth guard is no longer effective and how often to replace mouth guards have not yet been evaluated.

Studies that examine the effect of either mouth guard use directly or rule changes that mandate mouth guard use show that mouth guards can be effective at reducing the risk of dental injuries by 43% to 89% (**Table 2**).[49–52]

Despite the efficacy of wearing mouth guards and rules that enforce their use, many athletes choose not to wear mouth guards. Reasons for not using a mouth guard may include a lack of concern regarding injury risk, problems with speech, interference with breathing, or discomfort.[53–55] Players who reportedly always wear a mouth guard, even when it is not enforced, believe it protects them from injury and/or wear it out of habit.[54] It has been suggested that customized mouth guards that fit appropriately may be used more, lead to fewer complaints regarding sport performance being affected,[56,57] and may also provide superior protection. In a study of Australian football players, custom-fitted trilaminate mouth guards made from polyvinyl acetate polyethylene were associated with a 46% decrease in the risk of head and orofacial injuries compared with regular nonspecified mouth guards.[58]

HELMETS, HEADGEAR, AND FACE GUARDS

The protective effect of helmets, headgear, and face guards in reducing the risk of facial injuries has been examined in multiple sports.[59–62] Helmet design has improved because of standardization by testing organizations, including the National Operating Committee on Standards for Athletic Equipment (NOCSAE), the Canadian Standards Association, and the International Organization for Standardization.[63,64] For example, helmets in American football are required to have face guards that meet the NOCSAE standard.[63] Similarly, helmets in ice hockey are required to have face guards (either shield, cage, or combination type) that meet the relevant standard.[65–67] Other projectile sports also have standards for face guards: baseball,[68–70] cricket,[71,72] lacrosse,[73–75] and softball.[69,70]

Helmets and face guards have been effective at reducing the risk of facial injuries by 28% to 60%[59,60,62,76–78] and are effective in reducing, and in some cases eliminating, eye injuries (**Table 3**).[61,77,78]

The effectiveness of headgear to prevent facial injury has been mixed. Headgear in rugby union has been associated with nonsignificant reductions in superficial facial

Table 2
Studies examining the effectiveness of mouth guard use

Author and Year	Sport/Study Design/Years Studied/Country	Outcome (Injury Types Included)	Participants (Level, Sex, Age, Sample Size)	Intervention and Control Description	Reported IR (per 1000 h) or IP (per 100 Players)	Effect Estimates Reported or Calculated Based on Data Provided
Finch et al,[58] 2005	Australian Football League/ Group RCT/2001/ Australia	Head and orofacial injuries	Nonelite Men Divisions I, II, IV, seniors and juniors IG: n = 190, N = 12; mean age (SD) juniors = 23 y (3.0), mean age (SD) seniors = 26 y (2.7) CG: n = 111, N = 11; mean age (SD) juniors = 23 y (3.4), mean age (SD) seniors = 27 y (3.1)	IG: custom-made mouth guards (players were provided a trilaminate, polyvinyl acetate polyethylene mouth guard custom fitted by a dental technician) CG: usual mouth guard behavior	Head and orofacial injuries IG: IR, 1.8 injuries per 1000 exposure hours CG: IR, 4.4 injuries per 1000 exposure hours	Head and orofacial injuries Unadjusted IRR = 0.41 Adjusted IRR = 0.56 (0.32, 0.97) Covariates included division, age, BMI, previous injury, wore a mouth guard in the previous season (preseason risk-taking behavior score)
Labella et al,[49] 2002	Basketball/ Prospective cohort study/ 1999–2000/ United States	Oral soft tissue injuries, dental injuries, concussions	Collegiate men N = 50	IG: those wearing custom-fitted mouth guards CG: those not wearing mouth guards	Oral soft tissue injuries IG: 0.69 per 1000 AE CG: 1.06 per 1000 AE Dental injuries IG: 0.12 per 1000 AE CG: 0.67 per 1000 AE Concussions IG: 0.35 per 1000 AE CG: 0.55 per 1000 AE	Oral soft tissue injuries RRᵃ = 0.65 (0.23, 1.50) Dental injuries RRᵃ = 0.17 (0.004, 1.0) Concussion RRᵃ = 0.63 (0.12, 2.02)
Cohenca et al,[50] 2007	Basketball/ Historical cohort study/ 1996–2005/ United States	Dental trauma	Collegiate women 10 seasons IG: 12 athletes per season (72 athlete seasons) CG: 12 athletes per season (48 athlete season)	USC initiated a mouth guard mandate in 2000 IG: players playing with the mouth guard mandate 2000–2005 CG: players playing without the mouth guard mandate 1996–2000	Dental injuries IG: 2.8 per 100 athlete seasons CG: 8.3 per 100 athlete seasons	Dental injuries RRᵃ = 0.33 (0.03–2.33)

(continued on next page)

Table 2
(continued)

Author and Year	Sport/Study Design/Years Studied/Country	Outcome (Injury Types Included)	Participants (Level, Sex, Age, Sample Size)	Intervention and Control Description	Reported IR (per 1000 h) or IP (per 100 Players)	Effect Estimates Reported or Calculated Based on Data Provided
Quarrie et al,[51] 2005	Rugby union/ Ecological study/ 1995–2003/New Zealand	Dental trauma (measured using dental claims by insurance companies)	Male <19 y	In 1997 New Zealand introduced a mandatory mouth guard rule IG1: injury claims before the rule change CG1: injury claims after the rule change IG2: mouth guard wearers CG2: non–mouth guard wearers	NR	Rule change 43% reduction in claims between 1993 and 2003 Mouth guard wearers vs nonwearers RR[b] = 0.22 (0.18, 0.26)
Tanaka et al,[52] 2014	Rugby union/ Cross-sectional study/Japan	Oral injury	High school and medical school men High school: n = 69 age 17 ± 0.7 y (all custom-made mouth guards) Medical school n = 426, age = 22.5 y ± 2.6 y (85.2%) were custom made	IG: mouth guard use/ frequency of use in the fourth quartile as measured on a VAS CG: no mouth guard used/frequency of use in the first quartile as measured by VAS	Proportion of injuries sustained while not wearing a mouth guard High school: 14 out of 19 injuries Medical school: 121 out of 151 injuries	Oral injuries in fourth quartile of mouth guard use vs first quartile High school (<44% of the time vs >66% of the time) OR = 0.11 (0.02–0.66) Medical school (<5% of the time vs >82% of the time) OR = 0.27 (0.12–0.61)

Abbreviations: BMI, body mass index; NR, not reported; RCT, randomized controlled trial; USC, University of Southern California; VAS, visual analog scale.
[a] RR was calculated.
[b] RR was inversed.

injuries,[79] whereas boxing headgear has been found to significantly reduce the incidence of facial lacerations during bouts.[80–82] Soft-shell padded headgear can also be worn in soccer,[83] but has not been associated with a decrease in facial injuries.[84]

RULE CHANGES AND EDUCATION

Mouth guards, headgear, and eye protection have shown some effectiveness in reducing facial injuries; however, athletes may not be motivated to use protective equipment when it is optional for the sport. Rule changes that mandate protective equipment have been shown to be effective at increasing mouth guard use and eyewear protection, but not every rule change has been evaluated.[32,33,50,51] **Table 4** provides examples of some of the rule changes sport organizations have implemented to reduce injury.

Educational interventions may include pamphlets, television advertisements, workshops, or social media campaigns.[85] Educational and awareness campaigns have been used to promote greater use of protective equipment for sports without mandates for their use in place. For example, Eime and colleagues[37] examined squash players and their usage of appropriate protective eyewear when exposed to educational materials that encouraged their use. Those who had played in venues with educational materials on proper eyewear in squash were 2.4 times more likely to be wearing the proper protective eyewear than those who played in venues without such materials. Owners of venues that displayed educational materials on appropriate squash eyewear reported increased sales and rentals of protective eyewear. However, education regarding risks and provision of protective eyewear may not be enough to ensure continual use and consistent enforcement may be required. For example, in a randomized controlled trial including 60 youth basketball players (11–14 years old), both the intervention and control groups received an educational lecture on the risk of dental injuries and the benefits of mouth guard use.[55] Throughout the season the intervention group received verbal reinforcement to wear the mouth guard from the coach and study personnel, whereas the control group did not receive any such reinforcement. Following the 12-month study period, only 6 of 30 players (20%) not receiving reinforcement were still wearing their mouth guards regularly, whereas 23 of 30 players (77%) in the intervention group were.[55]

Educational material may influence behaviors related to facial injury protection for some people; however, such material has not been shown to prevent injuries. In a systematic review of educational interventions designed to prevent eye injury from both sport-related and non–sport-related activities, there was no evidence that educational interventions prevent eye injuries; however, they may influence knowledge and behavior.[85]

SPORT-SPECIFIC CONSIDERATIONS AND PREVENTION STRATEGIES
Badminton

Facial injuries in badminton can be a result of being hit by a racquet, another person, or with a shuttlecock. Given that the shuttlecock has a diameter of 18 mm, there is a risk that it can enter the eye.[21] Eye protection has been recommended to mitigate this risk but is not mandated or enforced, nor has it been evaluated.[92] Prescription glasses do not offer appropriate protection.[31] There is at least 1 reported case of prescription lenses shattering from the blow of a shuttlecock and resulting in a penetrating eye injury.[14] Badminton eye protection has the same recommended equipment standards as tennis, squash, and racquetball (AS/NZS [Australian/New Zealand Standard] 4006).[21]

Table 3
Summary of studies examining the effectiveness of helmets, headgear, and other facial protection

Author and Year	Sport/Study Design/Years Studied/Country	Outcome (Injury Types Included)	Participants (Level, Sex, Age, Sample Size)	Intervention and Control Description	Reported IR (per 1000 h) or IP (per 100 Players)	Effect Estimates Reported or Calculated Based on Data Provided
Danis,[59] 2000	Baseball/ Quasiexperimental study/1997/United States	Parent-reported facial injuries Player-reported facial injuries	IG: N = 136 teams, 743 athletes, 1214 parents CG: N = 102 teams, 1205 athletes, 988 parents	IG: supplied helmets with face guards and agreed to have all batters use a helmet with face guard for the season CG: voluntary use of helmet with face guard	Parent report of physician visits because of facial injury IG: 1.9 per 100 athletes CG: 2.7 per 100 athletes Player report of facial injury IG: 5.3 per 100 athletes CG: 4.1 per 100 athletes	Facial injuries reported by parents RR[a] = 0.72 (0.42–1.25) Facial injuries reported by the player RR[a] = 1.30 (0.83–2.0)
Marshall et al,[60] 2003	Baseball/Ecological study/1997–1999/ United States	Facial injury (eye, face, or nose)	Youth (aged 5–18 y)	IG: those wearing face guards CG: those not wearing face guards	Facial injury IG: 4.07 per 100,000 player-seasons CG: 2.42 per 100,000 player-seasons	Facial injury Adjusted RR = 0.65 (0.43–0.98) (adjusted for division)
Khan et al,[61] 2008	Hurling/Historical cohort/2003–2006/ Ireland	Eye injuries (hyphema, periorbital ecchymosis, retinal hemorrhage, commotion retinae, increased intraocular pressure, orbital fracture)	Youth (aged <18 y)	The Gaelic Athletic Association mandated full protective headgear for all players aged <18 y IG: eye injuries reporting at the emergency department after rule change CG: eye injuries reporting at the emergency department before rule change	IG: 2 injuries in hurling players aged <18 y after the rule change CG: 12 injuries in hurling players <18 y before the rule change	Significant reduction (χ^2 test, $P < .05$)

Study / Year	Design / Location	Injury type	Population	Intervention	Outcome measures	Results
Benson,[62] 1999	Ice hockey/Prospective cohort/1997–1998/Canada	Head and neck injury (including head and face injuries, neck injuries, and other injuries)	Canadian Inter-University Athletics Union, male, aged 18–29 y, n = 642, N = 22	Ontario Universities Athletic Association mandated full facial protection, whereas the Canadian West and Atlantic Universities Athletic Associations mandate, at minimum, half-visor protection IG: those wearing full-face shields CG: those wearing half-face visors	Head and face injuries IG: 1.41 per 1000 AE CG: 3.54 per 1000 AE Neck injuries IG: 0.29 per 1000 AE CG: 0.34 per 1000 AE Other injuries IG: 6.21 per 1000 AE CG: 7.53 per 1000 AE	Head and facial injuries RR = 0.40 (0.27–0.58) Neck injuries RR = 0.86 (0.32–2.33) Other injuries RR = 0.83 (0.83–1.02)
LaPrade et al,[76] 1995	Ice hockey/Prospective cohort/United States	Facial lacerations and neck injury	NCAA division 1, male	Mandatory use of face masks compared with a previous study in which face mask use was not mandatory IG: players with face mask mandate CG: players without the face guard mandate	Facial lacerations IG: 14.7–15.1 per 1000 player-game hours; 0.0–0.2 per 1000 player-practice hours CG: 21.8 per 1000 player-game hours; 0.6 per 1000 player-practice hours	Facial lacerations RR[a]: 0.67–0.69 (game play) RR[a]: 0.0–0.33 (practice play)

(continued on next page)

Table 3
(continued)

Author and Year	Sport/Study Design/Years Studied/Country	Outcome (Injury Types Included)	Participants (Level, Sex, Age, Sample Size)	Intervention and Control Description	Reported IR (per 1000 h) or IP (per 100 Players)	Effect Estimates Reported or Calculated Based on Data Provided
Stuart et al,[77] 2002	Ice hockey/Prospective cohort/United States	All facial injuries (including eye and neck)	Junior A, male, aged 16–21 y, n = 282, N = 10	IG: those wearing FFP CG: Those wearing PFP or NFP	All facial injury FFP: 23.2 per 1000 player-game hours PFP: 73.5 per 1000 player-game hours NFP: 158.9 per 1000 player-game hours Eye injury FFP: 0.0 per 1000 player-game hours[a] (ie, did not occur) PFP: 6.5 per 1000 player-game hours NFP: 30.6 per 1000 player-game hours	All facial injury RR: 0.46 (PFP vs NFP) RR: 0.15 (FFP vs NFP) RR: 0.32 (FFP vs PFP) Eye injury RR: 0.21 (PFP vs NFP) RR between FFP vs NFP and FFP vs PFP were unable to be calculated
Stevens et al,[78] 2006	Ice hockey/Prospective cohort/2001–2002/ North America	Facial injury (including nonconcussion head injury and eye injuries)	National Hockey League, male, n = 787	IG: those wearing PFP CG: those wearing NFP	NR/unable to be calculated	Nonconcussion head injury OR[a]: 0.18 (0.02–1.37) Eye injury OR: NA (OR unable to be calculated because of no cases of eye injury in those wearing visors)

Abbreviations: FFP, full facial protection; NA, not available; NFP, no facial protection; PFP, partial facial protection.
[a] RR was calculated.

Table 4
Examples of rule changes to reduce facial injuries

Year	Sport	Rule Change
2011[32,86]	Field hockey	NFHS mandated protective eyewear for women's field hockey players playing in NFHS-sanctioned competitions
1962[87]	Football	The NCAA mandated the use of mouth guards for all players at colleges and universities
2005[21,61]	Hurling	The Gaelic Athletic Association mandated full protective headgear for all players aged <18 y
2006[21,61]	Hurling	The Gaelic Athletic Association mandated full protective headgear for all players aged <21 y
2010[21,88–90]	Hurling	The Gaelic Athletic Association mandated full protective headgear for all players
1975	Ice hockey	The NCAA mandated the use of mouth guards that cover all the remaining teeth of 1 jaw for all players in colleges and university
1980	Ice hockey	Hockey Canada mandated facial protection certified by the Canadian Standard Association for all registered players
2013[91]	Ice hockey	NHL's Board of Governors approved a rule that mandated visors for new players who began playing in the 2013–2014 season
2005[21,33]	Lacrosse	US Lacrosse mandated protective eyewear for female high school lacrosse players
1997[51]	Rugby Union	New Zealand made mouth guards mandatory for all players aged <19 y during games
1998[51]	Rugby Union	New Zealand extended mandatory mouth guards to players of all levels of play during games
2003[51]	Rugby Union	New Zealand gave referees the power to eject players from the field if they are not wearing mouth guards appropriately

Baseball and Softball

Baseball has one of the highest risks of facial injuries in the United States in youth, with a high risk of eye injuries specifically.[4,15,21,93] Baseballs have a diameter of 73.8 mm and can be pitched at a velocity of more than 38 m/s.[21,94] A common cause of facial injuries is contact with the ball.[95,96] Facial injury prevention strategies for baseball include helmets with face guards; the use of safety balls; and the use of fitted mouth guards and eye protectors for batters, pitchers, and infielders.[95] Helmets with face guards (metal and plastic) have been shown to be effective at reducing the risk of facial and dental injuries in baseball by 35% to 37%.[59,60] The use of safety balls, which have a lower mass and less stiffness than a traditional baseball, has been shown to be effective in preventing injury in minor divisions (ages 7–12 years) and have been shown in a laboratory setting to reduce the likelihood of head and skull fractures.[60,97,98] Although concerns have been raised that the softness of safety balls could penetrate the orbit of the eye more deeply, causing more severe injury, this is only present in extremely soft balls and is less of a concern if safety balls and face guards meet safety standards.[99,100] Current safety standards for baseball include the ASTM F803 for all ages, ASTM F910 for youth, NOCSAE 072-04m13 for batters, and NOCSAE 024-11m13 for catchers.[21,68–70] Although most research has focused on baseball, many of the same safety recommendations for injury prevention are also applicable to softball.[21,22]

Basketball

In basketball, the most common causes for facial injuries include contact with another player or with the ball directly.[101] Basketball has been identified as being a high-risk sport for both eye[4,21,93,102] and dental injuries.[50,102] Although both eyewear and mouth guards have been recommended, prevention strategies have focused primarily on the use of mouth guards.[39,92] Mouth guard use has been associated with a 66% to 87% reduction in the risk of dental injuries in men and women playing collegiate basketball.[49,50] However, mouth guard use is not mandatory in most leagues and is limited across several countries.[101,103–105] Reasons basketball players cited for not wearing mouth guards include comfort, ignorance, nonavailability, and nonaffordability.[55,101,106] Coach reinforcement has been shown to be effective at encouraging mouth guard use in young basketball players when the league does not mandate it.[55]

Boxing

Mouth guards are the only protection equipment permitted at the international level in boxing. Amateur boxing headgear has been found to reduce the incidence of facial lacerations during bouts[80–82]; however, the Association Internationale de Boxe Amateur (AIBA) recently banned the use of soft-shelled padded headgear in selected amateur boxing competitions.[107] Boxing headgear is still used in training, with some models providing cheek coverage; however, no standards currently exist for boxing headgear.

Cricket

A cricket ball can travel at velocities of more than 28 m/s at the adult level and, along with the bails, pose significant risks of eye injuries.[21,108] Specifically, bails (the 2 pieces of wood that indicate when the stumps have been hit) pose a threat to the eyes of wicket keepers.[108] Furthermore, the sunglasses worn to avert glare are only designed to withstand 0.9 J of energy (vs squash or baseball eye protection, which is designed to withstand 16–19 J of energy).[21,108] In 2008, the England and Wales Cricket Board Science and Medicine Department initiated a project to identify the limitations of helmets and injury prevention in cricket. This project involved players, coaches, manufacturers, and administrators. Injury surveillance was initiated and identified more than 50 head injuries to batsman who were wearing helmets. The concerns they identified included the peak–face guard gap, overly flexible grilles, and players' modifications/fit. They developed an injury prevention plan that included 3 components: (1) an educational program for players to address risk perception about fit and choice, which included demonstrations of helmet failures leading to injury; (2) engagement with helmet manufactures, alerting them of injury problems and potential solutions; and (3) lobbying international organizations to improve helmet testing protocols.[109] There are now several standards for facial equipment in cricket. AS/NZS 4499 and BS7928 are designed to withstand the cricket ball (29.8–56.8 J), and BS7928-2 is designed for cricket wicketkeepers.[21]

Field Hockey

A field hockey ball weighs approximately 160 g and can reach speeds of 70 km/h or more. Combined with a 750-g stick, it is clear why it has been identified as having a high risk of eye injury.[21,53] A rule change mandating protective eyewear in women's high school field hockey was very effective at reducing eye injury, but this mandate has not extended to international level competition.[32] International field hockey players are only encouraged to wear shin, ankle, and mouth protection.[110] When not mandated, athletes do not always choose to wear mouth guards. In a survey of

110 female field hockey players in the United Kingdom, 42% wore mouth guards in games all the time.[53] Reasons for not using mouth guards included problems with speech (56%) or breathing (41%), or finding it uncomfortable (26%).[53]

Hurling and Camogie

Hurling and camogie both carry the risk of small projectiles and a stick that can come into close contact with other players. The balls weigh from 100 to 130 g and 90 to 110 g respectively, and can travel up to 150 km/h.[61] Camogie is played by women and is slightly different from hurling in that shoulder-to-shoulder contact is not permitted and the ball is slightly smaller. Prevention of facial injuries in hurling and camogie has largely been focused on the introduction of customized hurling helmets with face guards.[88] In 2010, the Gaelic Athletic Association mandated the use of hurling helmets with face guards that meet the standard (IS 355)[111] during training and games for all levels of hurling and camogie players.[112] Before the rule change, more than two-thirds (71%) of hurling players chose to wear helmets, most of which (88%) had face guards attached.[113] Similarly, three-quarters of camogie players chose to wear helmets, most of which (96%) had face guards. Since the introduction of helmets with face guards, the incidence of facial injuries in hurling has decreased.[114] However, serious eye injuries are still occurring because of modified or defective face guards.[89] One study recommended compulsory replacement of protective equipment every 5 years.[89]

Ice Hockey

Helmets in ice hockey are required to have face guards (shield, cage, or combination type) that meet the relevant standard.[65–67] Compared with no facial protection, full or partial protection significantly reduces the number and types of facial injuries in ice hockey.[76,77,115,116] However, full facial protection is superior to half facial protection in reducing the risk of head injury (excluding concussions), facial lacerations, and dental injuries,[62] and does not increase the risk of concussion or neck injury.[62,77,117] Because most high sticks have an upward trajectory, which can slip underneath a half-visor and strike the upper face and eye region, the half-visor may not adequately protect the upper face and periorbital region from catastrophic injury.[62,115] Further, full facial protection may also reduce concussion severity compared with a half-visor.[117] It has been recommended that all players should wear a certified helmet that is properly fitted and well secured so it protects from focal injury and from coming off during play.[118] In addition, mouth guards have been shown to prevent dental injuries and are recommended to be worn to protect the mouth, teeth, and jaw.[38,118–120] Although the use of a mouth guard may allow faster return to play following concussion,[117] the evidence is limited regarding the protective effect of mouth guards in reducing the risk of concussion.[121,122] Despite the protective benefits of wearing a mouth guard, many athletes are not routinely wearing them during competition.[40,123,124]

Mixed Martial Arts

Injury prevention strategies are challenging in the mixed martial arts. It has been noted that prevention strategies would be difficult to implement in a sport that openly promotes and awards victory and financial incentives for inflicting injury.[125] Although fighters are required to wear approved mouth guards and gloves,[126] fighting gloves may do little to reduce the accelerations that may produce injury.[127] Possible rule changes, such as stopping the fight for a 10-second countdown if a fighter is knocked down, may prevent further strikes to the face and also allow for the identification of a brain injury.[125] Referees should also be trained to better identify fighters who are defenseless and be able to stop the fight immediately.[125]

Rodeo

There is a paucity of research that has investigated the use of protective head gear in rodeo. Some evidence has suggested that bull riders who wear a helmet are at a reduced risk of head injury and facial fracture.[128,129] In addition, the authors and signatories of the Agreement Statement From the 1st International Rodeo Research and Clinical Care Conference agreed that the risks of bull riding without head protection far outweigh the risks of bull riding with head protection.[130] The high number of orofacial injuries in steer wrestlers suggests the need for mouth guard protection.[131,132]

Rugby Union, Rugby League, and Australian Football

Mouth guard use is strongly recommended by World Rugby[133] and national unions, such as those in Australia.[134] Mouth guards were made compulsory during matches and training for all rugby union players in New Zealand[135] after a study showed that compulsory mouth guard use was associated with a 43% reduction in rugby-related dental injury claims.[51] Despite recommendations and mandated use, players can choose not to wear mouth guards in training if rules are not enforced.[51,52,54] Reasons for not wearing mouth guards include that players find them uncomfortable or believe that it interferes with breathing.[54] Mouth guards have been found to prevent dental and orofacial injuries in rugby union players.[51,136–138] Similarly, mouth guards are commonly worn by approximately two-thirds of junior[139] and professional[54] rugby league players and have been found to prevent dental and orofacial injuries.[87]

Soft-shelled padded headgear is allowed to be worn in Australian football[140] and rugby league[141]; however, no standards currently exist.[142] World Rugby mandates design guidelines for headgear in rugby union[143]; however, facial coverage is minimized because of vision requirements. Headgear in rugby union has been associated with nonsignificant reductions in superficial facial injuries.[79]

Soccer

Despite the high prevalence of facial injuries in soccer, protective equipment is rarely used.[144] In a Canadian survey of adolescent soccer players conducted in 2006, 3.6% of players wore a mouth guard and 18% wore headgear. Eye protectors that meet the United States standard[26] are rarely seen in competition but have been found to prevent orbital intrusion in soccer and therefore reduce the likelihood of eye injury.[145,146] Soft-shell padded headgear can also be worn in soccer,[83] but has not been associated with a decrease in facial injuries.[84] Customized mouth guards may provide a good option for dental protection in soccer because communication is important. Compared with stock and boil-and-bite mouth guards, customized mouth guards allowed soccer players to speak, were much more comfortable, and did not affect breathing.[57] More research is needed to evaluate how the use of protection equipment can be promoted and evaluated in soccer.

Squash

Squash has been identified as having a moderate risk of both eye and dental injuries.[21,147] A squash ball has a diameter of 40 to 40.6 mm, weighs between 20 and 40 g, and can travel at speeds of 40 m/s.[21] Prevention of facial injuries in squash has largely focused on eye injuries and the use of protective eyewear. Although eye wear is generally recommended, different countries and associations have different rules regarding whether it is mandatory for players to use eye protection. For example, the use of protective eyewear is mandatory for all junior squash players in Australia, but not for adult squash players.[35] A survey conducted with 1163 adults in Australia in 2001 to 2002 found that 92.2% did not wear eyewear.[35] Reasons cited for squash players not wearing eyewear include that they did not want to (31.2%), it restricts vision (26.9%), they never thought about it (25.7%), it was not comfortable (23.9), there was no perceived risk (11.2%), prescription glasses were worn (10.4%), and the players did not like the look of them (5.6%).[35]

SUMMARY

There is some evidence that eye protection, mouth guards, helmets, and face guards are effective in reducing the risk of facial injury; however, such safety practices are not adopted universally by all athletes playing high-risk sports. Underlying beliefs about risk perception, comfort, ineffectiveness, utility, and a lack of awareness or enforcement have been identified as reasons people may not adopt preventive measures. There are methodological limitations in the studies evaluating protective equipment, such as lack of randomization of the intervention, inadequate follow-up period, inadequate controls, and lack of adjustment for sex and other potentially confounding variables. Randomization of equipment may present an ethical challenge and higher quality study designs, including controlling for confounding variables, could improve the quality of the literature evaluating prevention strategies for facial injury in sport. There are several high-risk sports that have not mandated or do not enforce the use of protective equipment. Valid evidence can assist with addressing the resistance caused by prevailing beliefs and could be essential in influencing rule changes.

REFERENCES

1. Arangio P, Vellone V, Torre U, et al. Maxillofacial fractures in the province of Latina, Lazio, Italy: Review of 400 injuries and 83 cases. J Craniomaxillofac Surg 2014;42(5):583–7.
2. Barrios J, Teuber C, Cosmelli R. Prevalence of sports-related maxillofacial fractures, at Clinica Alemana Santiago, Chile. Int J Oral Maxillofac Surg 2013; 42(10):1220.
3. Nardis A, da C, Costa SAP, et al. Patterns of paediatric facial fractures in a hospital of São Paulo, Brazil: a retrospective study of 3 years. J Craniomaxillofac Surg 2013;41(3):226–9.
4. Kim SH, Lee SH, Cho PD. Analysis of 809 facial bone fractures in a pediatric and adolescent population. Arch Plast Surg 2012;39(6):606.
5. Paes JV, de Sá Paes FL, Valiati R, et al. Retrospective study of prevalence of face fractures in southern Brazil. Indian J Dent Res 2012;23(1):80–6.
6. Muñante-Cárdenas JL, Olate S, Asprino L, et al. Pattern and treatment of facial trauma in pediatric and adolescent patients. J Craniofac Surg 2011;22(4):1251–5.
7. Chrcanovic BR, Abreu MHNG, Freire-Maia B, et al. Facial fractures in children and adolescents: a retrospective study of 3 years in a hospital in Belo Horizonte, Brazil. Dent Traumatol 2010;26(3):262–70.
8. Elhammali N, Bremerich A, Rustemeyer J. Demographical and clinical aspects of sports-related maxillofacial and skull base fractures in hospitalized patients. Int J Oral Maxillofac Surg 2010;39(9):857–62.
9. Calderoni DR, Guidi Mde C, Kharmandayan P, et al. Seven-year institutional experience in the surgical treatment of orbito-zygomatic fractures. J Craniomaxillofac Surg 2011;39(8):593–9.

10. Qing-Bin Z, Zhao-Qiang Z, Dan C, et al. Epidemiology of maxillofacial injury in children under 15 years of age in southern China. Oral Surg Oral Med Oral Pathol Oral Radiol 2013;115(4):436–41.

11. Leivo T, Haavisto A-K, Sahraravand A. Sports-related eye injuries: the current picture. Acta Ophthalmol 2015;93(3):224–31.

12. Armstrong GW, Kim JG, Linakis JG, et al. Pediatric eye injuries presenting to United States emergency departments: 2001–2007. Graefes Arch Clin Exp Ophthalmol 2013;251(3):629–36.

13. Yulish M, Reshef N, Lerner A, et al. Sport-related eye injury in northern Israel. Isr Med Assoc J 2013;15(12):763–5.

14. Ong HS, Barsam A, Morris OC, et al. A survey of ocular sports trauma and the role of eye protection. Cont Lens Anterior Eye 2012;35(6):285–7.

15. Pollard KA, Xiang H, Smith GA. Pediatric eye injuries treated in us emergency departments, 1990-2009. Clin Pediatr 2012;51(4):374–81.

16. Ain TS, Lingesha RT, Sultan S, et al. Prevalence of traumatic dental injuries to anterior teeth of 12-year-old school children in Kashmir, India. Arch Trauma Res 2016;5(1):e24596.

17. Stewart C, Kinirons M, Delaney P. Clinical audit of children with permanent tooth injuries treated at a dental hospital in Ireland. Eur Arch Paediatr Dent 2011; 12(1):41–5.

18. Mohajerani SH, Asghari S. Pattern of mid-facial fractures in Tehran, Iran. Dent Traumatol 2011;27(2):131–4.

19. Díaz JA, Bustos L, Brandt AC, et al. Dental injuries among children and adolescents aged 1-15 years attending to public hospital in Temuco, Chile. Dent Traumatol 2010;26(3):254–61.

20. Hecova H, Tzigkounakis V, Merglova V, et al. A retrospective study of 889 injured permanent teeth. Dent Traumatol 2010;26(6):466–75.

21. Dain SJ. Sports eyewear protective standards. Clin Exp Optom 2016;99(1): 4–23.

22. Committee on Sports Medicine and Fitness. American Academy of Pediatrics. Risk of injury from baseball and softball in children. Pediatrics 2001;107:782.

23. Standards Australia & Standards New Zealand. Eye protectors for racquet sports [amendment 1] AS/NZS 4066. Sydney (New South Wales): Standards Australia & Standards New Zealand; 1994.

24. Canadian Standards Association. Racquet sports eye protection CSA P400. Toronto: Canadian Standards Association; 1982.

25. British Standards Institution. Specification for eye-protectors for racket sports: squash BS 7930–1. London: British Standards Institution; 1998.

26. American Society of Testing and Materials. Standard specification for eye protectors for selected sports ASTM F803. West Conshohocken (PA): American Society of Testing and Materials; 2014.

27. Heimmel MR, Murphy MA. Ocular injuries in basketball and baseball: what are the risks and how can we prevent them? Curr Sports Med Rep 2008;7(5):284–8.

28. American Society for Testing and Materials. Standard specification for eye protectors for field hockey ASTM F2713. West Conshohocken (PA): American Society of Testing and Materials; 2014.

29. American Society of Testing and Materials. Standard specification for eye protectors for women's lacrosse ASTM F3077. West Conshohocken (PA): American Society of Testing and Materials; 2014.

30. Farrington T, Onambele-Pearson G, Taylor RL, et al. A review of facial protective equipment use in sport and the impact on injury incidence. Br J Oral Maxillofac Surg 2012;50(3):233-8.
31. Hoskin AK, Philip S, Dain SJ, et al. Spectacle-related eye injuries, spectacle-impact performance and eye protection. Clin Exp Optom 2015;98(3):203-9.
32. Kriz PK, Zurakowski RD, Almquist JL, et al. Eye protection and risk of eye injuries in high school field hockey. Pediatrics 2015;136(3):521-7.
33. Lincoln AE, Caswell SV, Almquist JL, et al. Effectiveness of the women's lacrosse protective eyewear mandate in the reduction of eye injuries. Am J Sports Med 2012;40(3):611-4.
34. Bro T, Ghosh F. Floorball-related eye injuries: the impact of protective eyewear. Scand J Med Sci Sports 2016. [Epub ahead of print].
35. Eime R, McCarty C, Finch CF, et al. Unprotected eyes in squash: not seeing the risk of injury. J Sci Med Sport 2005;8(1):92-100.
36. McLean CP, DiLillo D, Bornstein BH, et al. Predictors of goggle use among racquetball players. Int J Inj Contr Saf Promot 2008;15(3):167-70.
37. Eime R, Finch C, Wolfe R, et al. The effectiveness of a squash eyewear promotion strategy. Br J Sports Med 2005;39(9):681-5.
38. Tuna EB, Ozel E. Factors affecting sports-related orofacial injuries and the importance of mouthguards. Sports Med 2014;44(6):777-83.
39. American Dental Association. The importance of using mouthguards. J Am Dent Assoc 2004;135:1061.
40. Hawn KL, Visser MF, Sexton PJ. Enforcement of mouthguard use and athlete compliance in National Collegiate Athletic Association men's collegiate ice hockey competition. J Athl Train 2002;37(2):204-8.
41. American Dental Association. Athletic mouthguards acceptance program requirements. Chicago (IL): American Dental Association; 2016.
42. American National Standards Institute. Athletic mouth protectors and materials specification 99. New York: American National Standards Institute; 2013.
43. American Society for Testing and Materials. Standard practice for care and use of athletic mouth protectors ASTM F697. West Conshohocken (PA): American Society for Testing and Materials; 2016.
44. British Standards Institution. Mouthguards for use in sports and recreation [draft] BS 8563. London: British Standards Institution; 2011.
45. European Committee for Standardization. Mouthguards for use in sports [withdrawn] EN 15712. Brussels (Belgium): European Committee for Standardization; 2007.
46. Standards Australia. Guidelines for the fabrication, use and maintenance of sports mouthguards [withdrawn] HB 209-2003. Sydney (New South Wales): Standards Australia; 2003.
47. Gould TE, Piland SG, Shin J, et al. Characterization of mouthguard materials: thermal properties of commercialized products. Dent Mater 2009;25(12): 1593-602.
48. Rossi GD, Lisman P, Leyte-Vidal MA. A preliminary report of structural changes to mouthguards during 1 season of high school football. J Athl Train 2007;42(1): 47-50.
49. Labella CR, Smith BW, Sigurdsson A. Effect of mouthguards on dental injuries and concussions in college basketball. Med Sci Sports Exerc 2002;34(1):41-4.
50. Cohenca N, Roges RA, Roges R. The incidence and severity of dental trauma in intercollegiate athletes. J Am Dent Assoc 2007;138(8):1121-6.

51. Quarrie KL, Gianotti SM, Chalmers DJ, et al. An evaluation of mouthguard requirements and dental injuries in New Zealand rugby union. Br J Sports Med 2005;39(9):650–1.

52. Tanaka Y, Maeda Y, Yang T-C, et al. Prevention of orofacial injury via the use of mouthguards among young male rugby players. Int J Sports Med 2014;36(03): 254–61.

53. Hendrick K, Farrelly P, Jagger R. Oro-facial injuries and mouthguard use in elite female field hockey players. Dent Traumatol 2008;24(2):189–92.

54. Rayner W. Mouthguard use in match play and training in a cohort of professional rugby league players. Int J Sports Sci Coach 2008;3(1):87–93.

55. Spinas E, Aresu M, Giannetti L. Use of mouth guard in basketball: observational study of a group of teenagers with and without motivational reinforcement. Eur J Paediatr Dent 2014;15(4):392–6.

56. Duarte-Pereira DMV, Del Rey-Santamaria M, Javierre-Garces C, et al. Wearability and physiological effects of custom-fitted vs self-adapted mouthguards. Dent Traumatol 2008;24(4):439–42.

57. Queiróz AFVR, de Brito RB Jr, Ramacciato JC, et al. Influence of mouthguards on the physical performance of soccer players. Dent Traumatol 2013;29(6): 450–4.

58. Finch C, Braham R, McIntosh A, et al. Should football players wear custom fitted mouthguards? Results from a group randomised controlled trial. Inj Prev 2005; 11(4):242–6.

59. Danis RP. Acceptability of baseball face guards and reduction of oculofacial injury in receptive youth league players. Inj Prev 2000;6(3):232–4.

60. Marshall SW. Evaluation of safety balls and faceguards for prevention of injuries in youth baseball. JAMA 2003;289(5):568.

61. Khan MI, Flynn T, O'Connell E, et al. The impact of new regulations on the incidence and severity of ocular injury sustained in hurling. Eye (Lond) 2008;22(4): 475–8.

62. Benson BW. Head and neck injuries among ice hockey players wearing full face shields vs half face shields. JAMA 1999;282(24):2328.

63. National Operating Committee on Standards for Athletic Equipment. Standard method of impact test and performance requirements for football faceguards. Overland Park (KS): National Operating Committee on Standards for Athletic Equipment; 2015.

64. Echlin PS, Upshur REG, Peck DM, et al. Craniomaxillofacial injury in sport: a review of prevention research. Br J Sports Med 2005;39(5):254–63.

65. American Society for Testing and Materials. Standard specification for eye and face protective equipment for hockey players ASTM F513. West Conshohocken (PA): American Society for Testing and Materials; 2012.

66. American Society for Testing and Materials. Standard specification for head and face protective equipment for ice hockey goaltenders ASTM F1587. West Conshohocken (PA): 2012.

67. Canadian Standards Association. Face protectors for use in ice hockey CSA Z262.2. Toronto: 2015.

68. American Society of Testing and Materials. Standard specification for face guards for youth baseball ASTM F910. West Conshohocken (PA): 2015.

69. National Operating Committee on Standards for Athletic Equipment. Standard performance specification for newly manufactured baseball/softball batter's helmet mounted face protector. Overland Park (KS): 2013.

70. National Operating Committee on Standards for Athletic Equipment. Standard performance specification for newly manufactured baseball/softball catcher's helmet with faceguard. Overland Park (KS): 2013.
71. Standards Australia & Standards New Zealand. Protective headgear for cricket - faceguards AS/NZS 4499.3. Sydney (New South Wales): 1997.
72. British Standards Institution. Head and face protection for cricketers and face protectors for cricket wicket-keepers BS 7928-2. London: 2009.
73. Canadian Standards Association. Face protectors for use in lacrosse CSA Z262.8. Toronto: 2015.
74. National Operating Committee on Standards for Athletic Equipment. Standard performance specification for newly manufactured lacrosse helmets with face-guard. Overland Park (KS): 2012.
75. National Operating Committee on Standards for Athletic Equipment. Standard performance specification for newly manufactured lacrosse face protectors NOCSAE (ND)045-09m13. Overland Park (KS): National Operating Committee on Standards for Athletic Equipment; 2013.
76. LaPrade RF, Burnett QM, Zarzour R, et al. The effect of the mandatory use of face masks on facial lacerations and head and neck injuries in ice hockey. A prospective study. Am J Sports Med 1995;23(6):773–5.
77. Stuart MJ, Smith AM, Malo-Ortiguera SA, et al. A comparison of facial protection and the incidence of head, neck, and facial injuries in Junior A hockey players. A function of individual playing time. Am J Sports Med 2002;30(1):39–44.
78. Stevens ST, Lassonde M, de Beaumont L, et al. The effect of visors on head and facial injury in National Hockey League players. J Sci Med Sport 2006;9(3): 238–42.
79. Jones SJ, Lyons RA, Evans R, et al. Effectiveness of rugby headgear in preventing soft tissue injuries to the head: a case-control and video cohort study. Br J Sports Med 2004;38(2):159–62.
80. Jako P. Safety measures in amateur boxing. Br J Sports Med 2002;36(6):394–5.
81. Jákó P. Boxing. In: Kordi N, Maffuli N, Wroble RR, et al, editors. Combat sports medicine. London: Springer; 2009. p. 193–213.
82. Zazryn TR, McCrory PR, Cameron PA. Injury rates and risk factors in competitive professional boxing. Clin J Sport Med 2009;19(1):20–5.
83. Fédération Internationale de Football Association. Special medical protection items equipment regulations. Zürich (Switzerland): Fédération Internationale de Football Association; 2016. p. 48.
84. Delaney JS, Al-Kashmiri A, Drummond R, et al. The effect of protective head-gear on head injuries and concussions in adolescent football (soccer) players. Br J Sports Med 2008;42(2):110–5 [discussion: 115].
85. Shah A, Blackhall K, Ker K, et al. Educational interventions for the prevention of eye injuries. Cochrane Database Syst Rev 2009;(4):CD006527.
86. Kriz PK, Comstock RD, Zurakowski D, et al. Effectiveness of protective eyewear in reducing eye injuries among high school field hockey players. Pediatrics 2012;130(6):1069–75.
87. Knapik JJ, Marshall SW, Lee RB, et al. Mouthguards in sport activities: history, physical properties and injury prevention effectiveness. Sports Med 2007; 37(2):117–44.
88. Crowley PJ, Crowley MJ. Dramatic impact of using protective equipment on the level of hurling-related head injuries: an ultimately successful 27-year programme. Br J Sports Med 2014;48(2):147–50.

89. Kent D. Eye safety in hurling: a few remaining blind spots? Ir J Med Sci 2015; 184(3):707–11.

90. Ahern SE, Walker TWM, Sexton PFA, et al. A five year retrospective analysis of facial fracture pattern and aetiology of injury: do hurling helmets work? Ir J Med Sci 2012;181:S23.

91. Micieli JA, Zurakowski D, Ahmed K II. Impact of visors on eye and orbital injuries in the National Hockey League. Can J Ophthalmol 2014;49(3):243–8.

92. American Academy of Pediatrics. Committee on Sports Medicine and Fitness, American Academy of Ophthalmology, Eye Health and Public Information Task Force. Protective eyewear for young athletes. Ophthalmology 2004; 111(3):600–3.

93. Pieper P. Epidemiology and prevention of sports-related eye injuries. J Emerg Nurs 2010;36(4):359–61.

94. Urbin MA, Fleisig GS, Abebe A, et al. Associations between timing in the baseball pitch and shoulder kinetics, elbow kinetics, and ball speed. Am J Sports Med 2013;41(2):336–42.

95. Collins CL, Comstock RD. Epidemiological features of high school baseball injuries in the United States, 2005-2007. Pediatrics 2008;121(6):1181–7.

96. Bak MJ, Doerr TD. Craniomaxillofacial fractures during recreational baseball and softball. J Oral Maxillofac Surg 2004;62(10):1209–12.

97. King A, Hodgson V. Comparison of the effect of RIF and Major League Baseball impacts on the acceleration response and skull fracture patterns of cadaver heads. Tullahoma (TN): Worth Inc; 1992.

98. Viano DC, McCleary JD, Andrzejak DV, et al. Analysis and comparison of head impacts using baseballs of various hardness and a hybrid III dummy. Clin J Sport Med 1993;3(4):217–28.

99. Vinger P. Baseball eye protection: the effect of impact by major league and reduced injury factor baseball on currently available eye protectors. In: Hoerner EF, Cosgrove FA, editors. International Symposium on Safety in Baseball/Softball, 1995, Atlanta, GA. West Conshohocken (PA): ASTM; 1997. STP1313: 29–37.

100. Vinger PF, Duma SM, Crandall J. Baseball hardness as a risk factor for eye injuries. Arch Ophthalmol 1999;117(3):354–8.

101. Azodo CC, Odai CD, Osazuwa-Peters N, et al. A survey of orofacial injuries among basketball players. Int Dent J 2011;61(1):43–6.

102. Huffman EA, Yard EE, Fields SK, et al. Epidemiology of rare injuries and conditions among United States high school athletes during the 2005-2006 and 2006-2007 school years. J Athl Train 2008;43(6):624–30.

103. Keçeci AD, Eroglu E, Baydar ML. Dental trauma incidence and mouthguard use in elite athletes in Turkey. Dent Traumatol 2005;21(2):76–9.

104. Ma W. Basketball players experience of dental injury and awareness about mouthguard in China. Dent Traumatol 2008;24(4):430–4.

105. Perunski S, Lang B, Pohl Y, et al. Level of information concerning dental injuries and their prevention in Swiss basketball–a survey among players and coaches. Dent Traumatol 2005;21(4):195–200.

106. Spinas E, Savasta A. Prevention of traumatic dental lesions: cognitive research on the role of mouthguards during sport activities in paediatric age. Eur J Paediatr Dent 2007;8(4):193–8.

107. Association Internationale de Boxe Amateur. Interview with the AIBA Medical Commission Chairman. Boxing! AIBA Mag 2016;2–3.

108. Mann DL, Dain SJ. Serious eye injuries to cricket wicketkeepers: a call to consider protective eyewear. Br J Sports Med 2013;47(10):607–8.

109. Ranson C, Young M. Putting a lid on it: prevention of batting helmet related injuries in cricket. Br J Sports Med 2013;47(10):609–10.

110. The International Hockey Federation. Rules of hockey. Available at: http://www.fih.ch. Accessed May 18, 2016.

111. National Standards Authority of Ireland. Specification for helmets for hurling and camogie players IS 355. 2006. Available at: http://www.nsai.ie. Accessed May 1, 2016.

112. Gaelic Athletic Association. Rule 4-Equipment official guide - Part 2. Dublin (Ireland): Gaelic Athletic Association; 2015.

113. Hennessy B, Murray I, O'Connor K, et al. Prevailing attitude amongst current senior intercounty hurlers to head and facial protection: a pilot study. Ir J Med Sci 2007;176(4):279–81.

114. Murphy C, Ahmed I, Mullarkey C, et al. Maxillofacial and dental injuries sustained in hurling. Ir Med J 2010;103(6):174–6.

115. Bunn JW. Changing the face of hockey: a study of the half-visor's ability to reduce the severity of facial injuries of the upper-half of the face among east coast hockey league players. Phys Sportsmed 2008;36(1):76–86.

116. Stuart MJ, Smith A. Injuries in junior A ice hockey: a three-year prospective study. Am J Sports Med 1995;23(4):458–61.

117. Benson BW, Rose MS, Meeuwisse WH, et al. The impact of face shield use on concussions in ice hockey: a multivariate analysis. Br J Sports Med 2002;36(1):27–32.

118. Smith AM, Stuart MJ, Greenwald RM, et al. Proceedings from the Ice Hockey Summit on Concussion: a call to action. PM R 2011;3(7):605–12.

119. American Academy of Pediatric Dentistry. Policy on prevention of sports-related orofacial injuries. 2013. Available at: http://www.aapd.org/media/policies_guidelines/p_sports.pdf. Accessed May 1, 2016.

120. Newsome PR, Tran DC, Cooke MS. The role of the mouthguard in the prevention of sports-related dental injuries: a review. Int J Paediatr Dent 2001;11(6):396–404.

121. Benson BW, Hamilton GM, Meeuwisse WH, et al. Is protective equipment useful in preventing concussion? A systematic review of the literature. Br J Sports Med 2009;43(Suppl 1):i56–67.

122. Chisholm DA, Romanow NT, Schneider KJ, et al. Mouthguard use in youth ice hockey and the incidence of concussion and dental injuries [Abstract]. Clin J Sport Med 2015;25(1):0–3.

123. Duymus ZY, Gungor H, Erhan SE. Use of mouthguard rates among athletes during 2009 IIHF word U18 championship. Dentistry 2014;04(02). http://dx.doi.org/10.4172/2161-1122.1000195.

124. Berry DC, Miller MG, Leow W. Attitudes of Central Collegiate Hockey Association ice hockey players toward athletic mouthguard usage. J Public Health Dent 2005;65(2):71–5.

125. Hutchison MG, Lawrence DW, Cusimano MD, et al. Head trauma in mixed martial arts. Am J Sports Med 2014;42(6):1352–8.

126. Discover UFC. Championship UF. Rules and Regulations. Available at: http://www.ufc.ca/discover/sport/rules-and-regulations. Accessed May 25, 2016.

127. Schwartz ML, Hudson AR, Fernie GR, et al. Biomechanical study of full-contact karate contrasted with boxing. J Neurosurg 1986;64(2):248–52.

128. Brandenburg MA, Archer P. Survey analysis to assess the effectiveness of the bull tough helmet in preventing head injuries in bull riders: a pilot study. Clin J Sport Med 2002;12(6):360–6.

129. Brandenburg MA, Archer P. Mechanisms of head injury in bull riders with and without the Bull Tough helmet–a case series. J Okla State Med Assoc 2005; 98(12):591–5.

130. Andrews DM, Brett K, Bugg BH, et al. Agreement statement from the 1st International Rodeo Research and Clinical Care Conference. Clin J Sport Med 2005; 15(3):192–5.

131. Meyers MC, Laurent CM. The rodeo athlete: injuries - Part I. Sports Med 2010; 40(10):817–39.

132. Meyers MC, Laurent CM. The rodeo athlete: injuries - Part II. Sports Med 2010; 40(10):817–39.

133. World Rugby. Equipment, environment and emergency plan. Dublin (Ireland): World Rugby; 2016.

134. Australian Rugby Union. Australian rugby union medical and safety recommendations for players, coaches, administrators & match Officials. St Leonards (New South Wales): Australian Rugby Union; 2014.

135. New Zealand Rugby Players' Association. Collective agreement between New Zealand Rugby Union Incorporated and Rugby Players Collective Incorporated. Auckland (New Zealand): New Zealand Rugby Players' Association; 2013.

136. Ilia E, Metcalfe K, Heffernan M. Prevalence of dental trauma and use of mouthguards in rugby union players. Aust Dent J 2014;59(4):473–81.

137. Marshall SW, Loomis DP, Waller AE, et al. Evaluation of protective equipment for prevention of injuries in rugby union. Int J Epidemiol 2005;34(1):113–8.

138. Schildknecht S, Krastl G, Kuhl S, et al. Dental injury and its prevention in Swiss rugby. Dent Traumatol 2012;28(6):465–9.

139. Kroon J, Cox JA, Knight JE, et al. Mouthguard use and awareness of junior rugby league players in the Gold Coast, Australia. Clin J Sport Med 2016; 26(2):128–32.

140. Australian Football League. Law 9: Players' boots, jewellery and protective equipment. Docklands (Victoria): Australian Football League; 2016.

141. National Rugby League. Section 4: The players and players' equipment. New South Wales (Australia): 2013.

142. Patton DA, McIntosh AS. Considerations for the performance requirements and technical specifications of soft-shell padded headgear. Proc IMechE Part P: J Sports Engineering and Technology 2016;230(1):29–42.

143. World Rugby. Regulation 12. Schedule 1. Specifications relating to players' dress. Law 4 – players' clothing. Dublin (Ireland): World Rugby; 2015.

144. Correa MB, Knabach CB, Collares K, et al. Video analysis of craniofacial soccer incidents: a prospective study. J Sci Med Sport 2012;15(1):14–8.

145. Capao Filipe JA. Soccer (football) ocular injuries: an important eye health problem. Br J Ophthalmol 2004;88(2):159–60.

146. Vinger PF. The mechanism and prevention of soccer eye injuries. Br J Ophthalmol 2004;88(2):167–8.

147. Persic R, Pohl Y, Filippi A. Dental squash injuries - a survey among players and coaches in Switzerland, Germany and France. Dent Traumatol 2006;22(5): 231–6.

An Algorithmic Approach to Triaging Facial Trauma on the Sidelines

 CrossMark

Kristi Colbenson, MD

KEYWORDS

• Facial trauma in sports • Initial triage • Airway protection

KEY POINTS

- With any facial trauma, always complete a focused initial assessment following the ABC (airway, breathing, cervical spine) repeat ABCDE (airway, breathing, circulation, disability, exposure) mnemonic:
  - Airway: perform jaw thrust.
  - Breathing: facilitate clearance of secretions and assess for risk of aspiration.
  - Cervical spine: assess and immobilize athlete.
  - Airway: assess for 5 injuries that can lead to delayed airway obstruction.
  - Breathing: control aspiration risks and have a high index of suspicion for laryngeal trauma.
  - Circulation: manage epistaxis, transfer patient if posterior epistaxis is present, and obtain hemostasis of bleeding or perform compression and transfer patient.
  - Disability: determine Glasgow Coma Scale score and, if less than 15, continue to reassess; assess visual acuity and extraocular eye movements.
  - Exposure: reassess the cervical spine, transfer patient immediately if avulsed teeth are present, and examine for signs of basilar skull fracture or depressed skull fracture.
- The most critical component of the algorithm is the diagnosis and management of airway obstruction and aspiration.
- A thorough assessment will also include the recognition and treatment of associated high mortality injuries.

On the field, evaluation of facial trauma requires a focused initial assessment of the patient's airway and breathing, along with a good knowledge of the potential associated injuries. The resulting hemorrhage and deformity from facial trauma can distract providers from recognizing critical injuries that need immediate intervention; thus, it is important to stay true to a focused algorithm of evaluation. The algorithm to follow in facial trauma is the mnemonic ABC (airway, breathing, cervical spine), followed by a repeat ABCDE (airway, breathing, circulation, disability, exposure).

Mayo Clinic, 1216 2nd Street Southwest, Generose Building 410, Rochester, MN 55902, USA
E-mail address: Colbenson.kristina@mayo.edu

Clin Sports Med 36 (2017) 279–285
http://dx.doi.org/10.1016/j.csm.2016.11.003
0278-5919/17/© 2016 Elsevier Inc. All rights reserved.

AIRWAY

A good airway assessment is critical in the setting of facial injuries. Failure to recognize airway compromise and appropriately secure and protect the airway is the most common factor related to patient mortality in facial trauma.[1] Because facial injuries result from a significant impact, transient or prolonged loss of consciousness from intracranial injury can occur. When an athlete is unconscious, pharyngeal tone is lost, which can lead to airway obstruction by pharyngeal tissue, the tongue, mouth guards, and unstable fracture fragments. The initial airway assessment is focused on reversing this obstruction and assessing the athlete's ability to maintain airway patency. A modified jaw thrust is the first maneuver to perform to relieve airway obstruction (**Fig. 1**).

The modified jaw thrust is also a substantial pain generator, and if the athlete does not react, grimace, or reach toward the provider's hands, be concerned about the patient's neurologic ability to protect the airway. This maneuver requires a hard stop in the algorithm, and emergency medical services should be called because the patient is likely to require an airway intervention. Airway intervention in facial trauma is difficult and should only be attempted by experienced providers. Temporizing measures include continuing a modified jaw thrust to allow ventilation, and, should the patient become apneic or require positive pressure ventilation, a bag mask valve can be used to provide oxygenation. It may be difficult to obtain a good seal on the bag mask valve and appropriately oxygenate the athlete because of the unstable nature of the facial injuries. However, multiple supraglottic airway devices exist to maintain airway patency for oxygenation in these situations (**Fig. 2**).

However, these measures are only temporizing, because hemorrhage and vomitus can still obstruct the airway. Therefore, it is critical to recognize the potential for airway compromise and arrange the patient's transfer to the nearest emergency department to achieve a definitive airway. If the patient is conscious and can clear secretions by providing a cough reflex, progress immediately to step B.

BREATHING

Hemorrhage, vomitus, and secretions associated with facial injuries can lead to aspiration and hypoxia, so initial assessment is focused on the patient's ability to produce

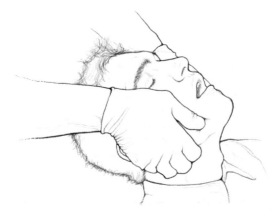

Fig. 1. Modified jaw thrust. Place 2 fingers superior and posterior to the angle of the mandible in the soft spot anterior to the mastoid process. Pull forward on the mandible to relieve airway obstruction. This maneuver is modified such that it does not involve manipulation of the cervical spine. (*Courtesy of* the Mayo Clinic Foundation, Rochester, MN; with permission.)

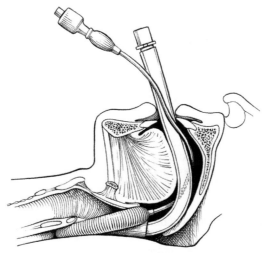

Fig. 2. Supraglottic devices such as a laryngeal mask airway (shown), esophageal tracheal double-lumen airway (Combitube; Covidien), and disposable supraglottic airway (King Systems) can serve as a provisional means of maintaining airway patency to allow oxygenation. Placement of these devices requires minimal training, and they are simple and efficient to use. (*Courtesy of* the Mayo Clinic Foundation, Rochester, MN; with permission.)

a good cough reflex and clear secretions. Athletes who, because of altered mental status, are unable to clear secretions need to immediately be placed in a position to allow clearance, either side lying or upright. However, before positioning a patient to an upright and forward-leaning position, step C must be assessed.

CERVICAL SPINE

The first step should be to feel for a carotid pulse in a minimally responsive athlete after trauma, but facial injury leads to hypoxia, not acute cardiovascular collapse. Therefore, C in this algorithm stands for cervical spine. Up to 10% of facial trauma is complicated by cervical spine injury.[2] Providers must immediately assess the patient for cervical spine tenderness. Midline cervical spine tenderness, bilateral paresthesias or weakness, and/or alteration in mental status require immediate on-field cervical spine stabilization.

Once the initial assessment of airway, breathing, and cervical spine tenderness is addressed, a good initial triage reassesses and considers more subtle findings that can imminently threaten the athlete's safety: ABCDE.

AIRWAY 2

Airway obstruction may not be immediately recognizable; thus, reassessment is vital. If there are findings concerning for a cervical spine injury in a helmeted athlete, maintain good spinal precautions with the helmet on, but gain access to the airway by removing the face mask. Several specific injuries must be assessed[3] because they can lead to delayed airway compromise:

1. Mandible fractures: bilateral anterior mandible fractures can cause the fractured symphysis and the tongue base to prolapse posteriorly, obstructing the oropharynx.
2. Le Fort fractures: posterior and inferior displacement of a fractured maxilla can block the nasopharyngeal airway; it can also lead to massive hemorrhage from an injured maxillary artery, causing aspiration.

3. Foreign bodies: fractured teeth, bone fragments, mouth guards, and debris may block the airway anywhere along the oropharynx and larynx. The athlete should attempt to expel foreign bodies through coughing or nose blowing. In unconscious patients, a provider should not perform a blind finger sweep in the oropharynx, given the potential for pushing the obstruction deeper. Instead, foreign bodies should be removed by using suction or forceps.
4. Soft tissue swelling: swelling within the oropharynx and larynx may cause delayed airway compromise. Be aware of the potential for this, which presents as the development of an inspiratory wheeze that suggests narrowing of the upper airway.
5. Trismus, decreased mouth opening from underlying muscle spasm or fracture, in the setting of associated hemorrhage or oropharyngeal swelling creates a difficult airway situation. The presence of trismus requires immediate transfer to the nearest emergency department because the options for airway intervention become exceptionally limited.

If a provider is concerned for any of these situations, emergency medical services must be called, a modified jaw thrust should be maintained, and the providers should prepare to appropriately maintain patency of the airway, as described in the initial airway assessment.

BREATHING 2

Providers should continue to monitor the athlete for aspiration risks by assessing the athlete's ability to clear secretions and blood from the nares and oropharynx. Specific attention should be paid to signs of posterior epistaxis. Posterior nosebleeds are often of arterial origin, can lead to profuse bleeding down the back of the throat, and can present a serious risk of airway compromise from aspiration of blood. If there is concern for posterior epistaxis, the patient must be placed in the side-lying or upright position bent forward.

A commonly overlooked injury associated with facial injury is laryngeal trauma that subjects the athlete to airway obstruction and compromises the ability to oxygenate and ventilate. It is vital to maintain a high index of suspicion for laryngeal trauma; missing it can be life threatening, with mortality as high as 40%.[4] Specific physical examination findings to be aware of include hoarseness, dyspnea, stridor, subcutaneous emphysema, and loss of anatomic landmarks in the neck.[5] There is no clear correlation between the extent of the underlying injury and the patient's presenting symptoms, so if any of the symptoms discussed earlier are present, immediate transfer to the nearest emergency department must be arranged because a surgical airway or fiberoptic intubation are the only ways to secure the patient's airway.[6]

CONTROL HEMORRHAGE

Epistaxis and hemorrhage from highly vascularized facial tissue can lead to considerable blood loss and can put the patient at risk for aspiration; thus, controlling hemorrhage is vital in the initial triage of facial injuries. The most common type of epistaxis is an anterior nosebleed. Acute management consists of having the patient blow the nose and expel any clots, followed by administration of a local vasoconstriction agent such as oxymetazoline (Afrin; Bayer), then immediate uninterrupted compression for 15 minutes distal to the nasal septum. However, this does not address posterior epistaxis, and these patients will continue to have bleeding down the back of the oropharynx. As already discussed, posterior nosebleeds are of particular concern because of the potential for significant hemorrhage from an arterial source. The only

option for controlling a posterior nosebleed is posterior packing, which is contraindicated in the setting of facial trauma, because a skull base fracture poses an inherent
risk for the inadvertent intracranial placement of packing material or devices. Even if
the provider is not concerned for underlying skull base fractures, posterior packing
in the training room or on the field should be done with extreme caution. Posterior
packing requires sedation and can cause substantial bradycardia. Athletes who
have symptoms of a posterior nosebleed should be placed in the upright forward-
leaning position and transfer arranged to the nearest emergency department.

Extensive arterial hemorrhage from facial wounds can occur with injury to the maxillary artery, the superficial temporal artery, or the angular artery. For facial lacerations,
the initial step is compression, followed by infiltration of lidocaine with epinephrine to
promote local vasoconstriction. If the source of bleeding is easily identifiable and not
controlled, a temporary figure-of-eight suture can be used to ligate the bleeding vessel.

In facial injury, it is exceptionally important to not just blindly place clamps in the
hopes of obtaining hemostasis, because this can lead to facial nerve paralysis. If hemorrhage cannot be controlled through the previous methods, place a compressive
facial dressing and transfer the athlete to the nearest emergency department.

DISABILITY

Up to 23% of facial fractures are associated with an underlying head injury; thus, the patient's neurologic status must be assessed to identify those at risk for mental status
decline and those who may require emergency transfer for further imaging and work-up.[7]

The Glasgow Coma Scale (GCS) (**Table 1**) is a neurologic scale that can quickly be
used as an objective evaluation tool to continually assess a patient's neurologic status. The patient's motor, verbal, and eye responses are evaluated, with points given
corresponding with the achieved response, and the 3 numbers totaled to arrive at a
GCS score (range, 3–15). Patients with GCS scores less than 8 require emergent intubation, and those with GCS scores less than 15 require reassessment. If at 2 hours
postinjury the athlete continues to have a GCS score less than 15, the patient should
be transferred to an emergency department for head computed tomography (CT). This
recommendation is in accordance with a powerful clinical decision tool, the Canadian
Head CT Rule,[8] which showed that a GCS score less than 15 more than 2 hours after
injury was 100% sensitive for head injuries requiring neurosurgical intervention.

Ocular injury is highly associated with facial trauma, so providers must perform
an initial triage of the patient's ocular disability. Visual acuity is the vital sign of the
eye and must be assessed. If there is a change in visual acuity in 1 or both eyes, the provider must first screen for the presence of an open globe injury (presentation and management are discussed elsewhere). An open globe is a medical emergency that requires
immediate transfer to the nearest emergency department. Before transfer, loosely cover
the affected eye and treat the patient for potential nausea. The other ocular disability to
document is extraocular eye movements. Deficits in full range of extraocular eye movements can suggest an underlying orbital fracture complicated by muscle entrapment or
orbital compartment syndrome. These injuries require emergent work-up and intervention,[9] especially given the potential for stimulation of the oculocardiac reflex associated
with these injuries. This reflex can cause concerning arrhythmias; most commonly bradycardia but also atrioventricular block, ventricular tachycardia, and asystole.

EXPOSURE

The final step in the algorithm is to fully expose the patient and assess for associated
injuries. Cervical spine injury has the highest correlation with facial trauma, and it is

Table 1
The Glasgow Coma Scale

Response		Points				
	1	2	3	4	5	6
Motor	Makes no movements	Extension to painful stimuli	Flexion to painful stimuli	Withdrawal to painful stimuli	Localizes painful stimuli	Obeys commands
Verbal	Makes no sounds	Incomprehensible sounds	Utters inappropriate words	Confused, disoriented	Oriented, converses normally	
Eyes	Does not open eyes	Opens eyes in response to painful stimuli	Opens eyes in response to voice	Opens eyes spontaneously		

imperative to reassess the athlete's cervical spine for any midline tenderness or neurologic deficit that requires emergent evaluation and stabilization. Other high-risk injuries to specifically assess include skull fractures that carry a high probability of associated intracranial bleeding, such as an open or depressed skull fracture or a basilar skull fracture. Signs of a basilar skull fracture include hemotympanum, raccoon eyes, battle sign, or cerebrospinal fluid rhinorrhea. These injuries require emergent transfer of the athlete for imaging and evaluation. The final step in exposure is to assess the athlete's dentition. Specifically, providers must count the athlete's teeth and assess for tooth stability and tooth subluxation. A tooth avulsion or subluxation is a dental emergency that requires emergent reimplantation and stabilization.

Facial injuries are common in sports and can be associated with airway compromise, aspiration, and hemorrhage. It is critical to not be distracted by the patient's pain, deformity, or bleeding and miss associated injuries that have a high mortality risk. With any facial trauma, always complete a focused initial assessment by following the ABC repeat ABCDE mnemonic:

- Airway: perform jaw thrust.
- Breathing: facilitate clearance of secretions and assess for risk of aspiration.
- Cervical spine: assess and immobilize athlete.
- Airway: assess for 5 injuries that can lead to delayed airway obstruction.
- Breathing: control aspiration risks and have a high index of suspicion for laryngeal trauma.
- Circulation: manage epistaxis, transfer patient if posterior epistaxis is present, and obtain hemostasis of bleeding or perform compression and transfer patient.
- Disability: determine GCS score and, if less than 15, continue to reassess; assess visual acuity and extraocular eye movements.
- Exposure: reassess the cervical spine, transfer patient immediately if avulsed teeth are present, and examine for signs of basilar skull fracture or depressed skull fracture.

REFERENCES

1. Gruen RJ, Jurkovich GJ, McIntyre LK, et al. Patterns of errors contributing to trauma mortality: lessons learned from 2,594 deaths. Ann Surg 2006;244:371–80.
2. Haug RW, Wible RT, Likavec MJ, et al. Cervical spine fractures and maxillofacial trauma. J Oral Maxillofac Surg 1991;49:725.
3. Hutchinson IL, Lawlor M, Skinner D. ABC of major trauma. Major maxillofacial injuries. BMJ 1990;301:595–9.
4. Atkins BZ, Abbate S, Fisher SR, et al. Current management of laryngotracheal trauma: case report and literature review. J Trauma 2004;56:185–90.
5. Kim JP, Cho SJ, Son HY, et al. Analysis of clinical feature and management of laryngeal fracture. Yonsei Med J 2012;53:992–8.
6. Paluska SA, Lansford CD. Laryngeal trauma in sport. Curr Sports Med Rep 2008; 7(1):16–21.
7. Zandi M, Seyed Hoseini SR. The relationship between head injury and facial trauma: a case-control study. Oral Maxillofac Surg 2013;3(17):201–7.
8. Stiell IG, Wells GA, Vandemheen K, et al. The Canadian CT Head Rule for patients with minor head injury. Lancet 2001;357(9266):1391–6.
9. Sugamata A, Yoshizawa N, Shimanaka K. Timing of operation for blowout fracture with extraocular muscle entrapment. J Plast Surg Hand Surg 2013;47:454–7.

Facial Injuries in Sports, Soft Tissue Injuries (Abrasions, Contusions, Lacerations)

Guy L. Lanzi, DMD*

KEYWORDS

- Facial injury • Sports • Soft tissue • Treatment

KEY POINTS

- Soft tissue injuries can be grouped generally into three categories: contusions, abrasions, and lacerations.
- All open wounds of the face need to be cleansed and explored to assess severity and potential related injury.
- Most frequently complications involve infection, scar formation, compromise of function and rarely, missed injury.
- Infection is addressed with debridement and incision and drainage as needed, and addition or substitution of appropriate antibiotics.
- Scar revision if necessary should be done generally after the scar is mature and preferably in the "off season".

Despite adequate oral-facial protection, soft tissue injuries occur regularly in sports. In certain sports, like professional ice hockey, the face and mouth are more vulnerable. No sport has shown the value of protection in reducing the frequency and severity of these injuries more than hockey. Mandatory institution of face shields in the American Hockey League all but eliminated eye injuries and, anecdotally, there are fewer facial lacerations at the collegiate level, where cages are required, than at the National Hockey League level. However, soft tissue injuries still occur. Their accurate diagnosis, including collateral damage, and prompt treatment are critical not only in terms of return-to-play issues but also to achieve ultimate optimal functional and esthetic results.

As with all sports-related trauma, before specific diagnoses and treatments are rendered general assessment must be performed and other more serious injuries ruled out, as described previously. Because of the proximity of the face to the brain, cervical spine, and airway, suspicion for related trauma must be high, initially ruled out, and followed for late or occult injury for an appropriate length of time.[1]

Disclosures: None.
Department of Surgery, Cooper University Hospital, Camden, NJ, USA
* 15 East Euclid Avenue, Haddonfield, NJ 08033.
E-mail address: rollcast2@yahoo.com

CONTUSIONS

Soft tissue injuries can be grouped generally into 3 categories: contusions, abrasions, and lacerations. Contusions or bruises are the simplest and most common soft tissue injury. They generally result from blunt force trauma, and can occur from many mechanisms, including collision or fall; contacts with equipment, including sticks or bats, or fixed equipment, including helmets, guards, pads, or footwear; or from strikes from game-related projectiles. Minor bruises require no significant acute treatment other than ice and often do not interfere with return to play. Postactivity ice and rest are generally adequate. More severe contusions may involve underlying soft and hard tissue injuries. Soft tissue injuries can include nerve or vascular trauma, and temporary altered sensation and hematomas are the most likely sequelae. Motor nerve injury is rare but may occur. Nerve contusions generally resolve spontaneously with ice and time. Ice and electrical stimulation and warm compresses may assist along with massage or physical therapy for more prolonged effects. Hematomas generally resolve spontaneously as well but caution must be taken with expanding hematomas, especially around the airway. (Nasal septal and ear hematomas are addressed elsewhere in this issue.) Hematomas of the masseter or temporalis muscles may cause trismus. Hemarthrosis of the temporomandibular joint can occur with jaw contusion and may cause trismus as well. Rest and a soft diet can aid in treatment. Hematomas respond well to warm compresses, and secondary infection of closed hematomas is rare. Intraoral inspection after facial contusion is important to rule out intraoral laceration secondary to blunt trauma from mouth guards, dental appliances, or teeth. Orthodontic hardware (braces), especially in teens but increasingly in adults, is notorious for causing serious mouth injuries after simple contusions.[2]

Hard tissue injuries to teeth and to bones can also occur with contusion; the more severe the contusion the higher the index of suspicion should be, and diagnosis and treatment of these collateral injuries are discussed in depth elsewhere. Two to especially watch out for are the Battle sign, which indicates basilar skull fracture, and so-called raccoon eyes, which indicate midface fractures[3] (**Fig. 1**).

ABRASIONS

Abrasions are superficial injuries to the skin no deeper than the epidermis, and bleeding, if present, is minimal. Minor abrasions generally do not scar but deeper abrasions generally bleed and may scar. It is important to understand that even the most minor abrasion is contaminated and may become infected. They are susceptible to tetanus and to methicillin-resistant *Staphylococcus aureus*, particularly if in contact with field dirt or colonized athletic padding. Tetanus toxoid status should be checked and systemic antibiotics should be considered when appropriate. Like contusions, abrasions rarely affect immediate return to play but abrasions generally should be cleansed and dressed at the appropriate time and protected from reinjury, especially if there is danger of repeated contact with clothing or protective gear.

As in the case of contusion, return to play is generally guided by the athlete's comfort level. The hallmark of treatment of abrasions is cleansing and debridement, especially of dirt or other contaminants. In the absence of allergies, antibiotic ointment can be applied and, especially for more extensive abrasions, a covering dressing is beneficial. This dressing can be either tape and gauze, commercial adhesive bandage, or even bio-occlusive dressings like Tegaderm. Skin adhesives like Mastisol or tincture of benzoin can help dressings adhere to sweat-drenched athletes. Extensive or deep abrasions tend to develop early cicatrix, which can lead to scarring. Daily debridement of scabbing with gauze and hydrogen peroxide, and reapplication of antibiotic ointment, can significantly reduce scar formation. Prevention of infection is key, especially in deep abrasion.

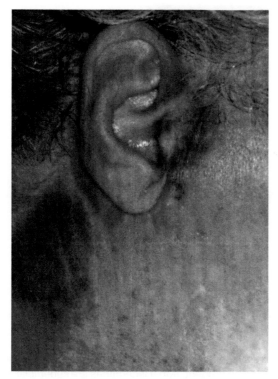

Fig. 1. Battle sign.

Appropriate use of systemic antibiotics may be indicated and good hygiene practice is vital to help reduce contamination and especially more serious MRSA infection.

Facial abrasions should be cleaned and debrided and dressed at least once a day to reduce infection and scarring (**Fig. 2**).

FACIAL LACERATIONS

Facial lacerations are the most variable of the soft tissue injuries that athletes can sustain. They can be caused by blunt or sharp trauma, they can occur intraorally and extraorally, and they can vary from a superficial skin nick to a through-through lip laceration or deep facial laceration involving significant vascular disruption or injury to collateral vital structures. There are natural skin tension lines in the face. Lacerations parallel to these lines are less likely to cause widened scars than incisions that are perpendicular to these lines.

Lacerations perpendicular to skin tension lines are more likely to cause widened scars. Steri-Strips after suture removal help greatly (**Fig. 3**).

GENERAL PRINCIPLES

All open wounds of the face need to be cleansed and explored to assess severity and potential related injury. Because of the rich blood supply to the face, hemostasis is always a prime concern of initial treatment. Initial hemostasis is best achieved with direct pressure, whether with a gauze pad or a towel. Hemostatic agents like Surgicel packed into the wound can assist in achieving an initial clot. Brisk arterial bleeding of a facial or neck vessel can be life threatening and prompt application of pressure, triage, and transport to the hospital is sometimes the necessary option. Similarly, brisk

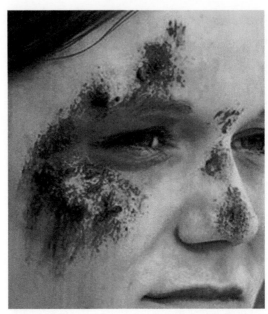

Fig. 2. Facial abrasions should be cleaned and debrided and dressed at least once a day to reduce infection and scarring.

bleeding into the airway can be uncomfortable or even dangerous, and speedy triage and transport may also be prudent. (Most lacerations are superficial and do not pose a problem for hemostasis and acute treatment.)

Wounds then need to be inspected for possible collateral injuries and foreign bodies. Other structures that can be injured with lacerations include nerves (facial and trigeminal), salivary ducts (parotid or submandibular), and lacrimal apparatus. In addition, there may be concomitant hard tissue injury to underlying bone or to the dentition. Lacerations to, or close to, bone should be inspected for fracture. Similarly, lacerations near the dentition, and in particular intraoral lacerations, need to be explored for dental injuries or fractures. Fractured teeth are commonly associated with lacerations, and wounds need to be explored in turn for tooth fragments or fragments of dental fillings or appliances (**Figs. 4** and **5**).

ANESTHESIA

Anesthesia can be provided by topical, local infiltration, or regional block. Amide anesthetics (eg, lidocaine, bupivacaine, mepivacaine) are used most commonly. Allergic reactions are uncommon and are usually related to the preservatives. Anesthetics with epinephrine generally last longer and give the added effect of bleeding control. When using anesthetics containing epinephrine care should be taken to avoid areas with end arteries (eg, nasal tip). In the face, this effect is usually overcome by the extensive blood supply.

Applicable regional blocks and the area of anesthesia (**Fig. 6**A, B):

- Supraorbital and supratrochlear block: forehead, anterior one-third of the scalp
- Infraorbital block: lower lid, upper lid, and lateral aspect of the nose
- Mental nerve block: lower lip and chin

(Mental and infraorbital blocks can be given intraorally)

- Inferior alveolar nerve block: lower lip, chin, tongue, teeth, and mucosa (**Fig. 6**C)

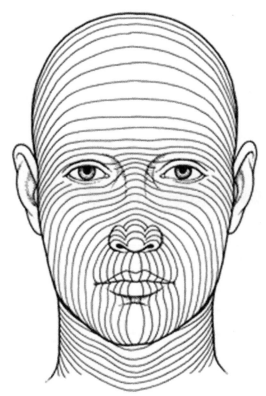

Fig. 3. Lacerations perpendicular to skin tension lines are more likely to cause widened scars. Steri-Strips after suture removal help greatly.

- Long buccal nerve block: cheek and alveolar mucosa
- Lingual nerve block: tongue and floor of mouth

TREATMENT
Simple Lacerations

Cleanse, as needed, then sterile prep. If return to play is an issue, sutures are recommended, although Steri-Strips and Mastisol or surgical adhesives can be used for temporary closure until there is an opportunity to place sutures. If return to play is not an issue, particularly with children, Steri-Strips and Mastisol or surgical adhesives provide excellent options. Regardless of which is used, the wound edges are approximated and closed. If strips are used, generally 3-mm (0.125″) or 6.0-mm (0.25″) strips are adequate, and Mastisol helps them remain in place. If surgical cyanoacrylate adhesive is used, the wound is approximated and several layers are applied, allowing each layer to dry before applying the next. Care must be taken around the eyes or lips. If the wound requires sutures, a 5-0 nonresorbable suture like nylon or proline is preferred for most of the face, with 6-0 nylon or proline for eyelids and 3-0 or 4-0 silk or nylon for the scalp.[4]

Deeper skin or scalp lacerations require more complex, layered closures. Layered closures allow better approximation of like tissues (muscle, subcutaneous tissue); eliminate dead space and reduce infection; improve the ultimate scar and function; and allow a better, more tension-free closure. For deeper layers, including periosteal, deep muscle, or galea, 4-0 undyed Vicryl on an appropriate-sized cutting needle (generally P3 or PS2 for scalp) is recommended. Subcutaneous closure is generally

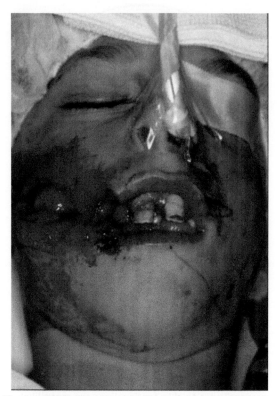

Fig. 4. Deep facial lacerations like this must be explored for collateral injury: in this case, parotid duct and facial nerve.

done with 4-0 chromic gut also on a cutting P3 or PS2 needle. Deep and subcutaneous sutures are generally placed in reverse fashion to bury the knot, and are generally placed in interrupted fashion. Then the skin is closed with interrupted 5-0 nylon or proline as in simple lacerations. A running stitch can be used for the skin, especially if subcutaneous closure has left the skin well approximated. However, interrupted skin sutures give more control if the skin edges are at slightly different levels. Alternatively a subcuticular running closure can be performed with a resorbable suture like

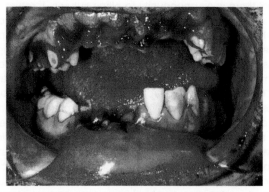

Fig. 5. Intraoral lacerations with obvious dental injury and missing teeth require that the wound and airway be carefully inspected for foreign bodies.

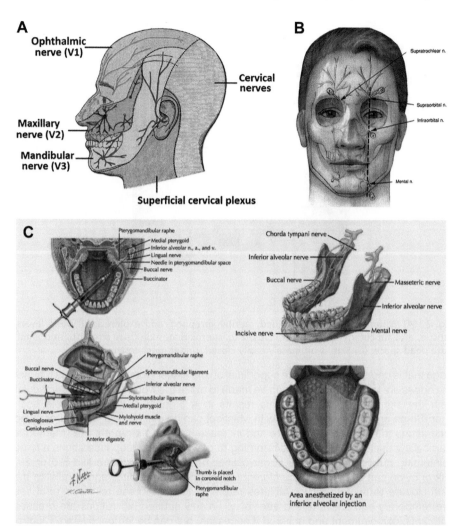

Fig. 6. (*A*) Dermatomes divisions of trigeminal nerve. (*B*) Facial regional blocks. (*C*) Inferior alveolar nerve block. a., artery; n., nerve; v., vein. ([*C*] Copyright © 2016. Used with permission of Elsevier. All rights reserved. www.netterimages.com.)

Monocryl. Hemostasis for deeper wounds is achieved with pressure, electrocautery, hemostats, surgical ties, or well-placed deep sutures (**Fig. 7**).

Most sports-related lacerations are caused by blunt trauma, and result in burst-type open wounds, often with jagged irregular edges (the exception to this is a hockey skate cut laceration, which is more like a surgical incision). If there are grossly jagged edges, plastic closure can often be facilitated by sharp judicious trimming of the wound edges with a knife or scissors. Trimming should not be extensive; matching irregularities in the edges of the skin wound can help in properly approximating the skin, much like fitting together the pieces of a jigsaw puzzle, but small tissue tags, and especially potential necrotic tissue, should be trimmed.[5]

Layered closure is invaluable when the wound is tangential, as many are, because the deeper layer closure can help level a tangential wound so that the skin edges are ultimately level. To level a tangential wound the suture bite is deeper on the wound

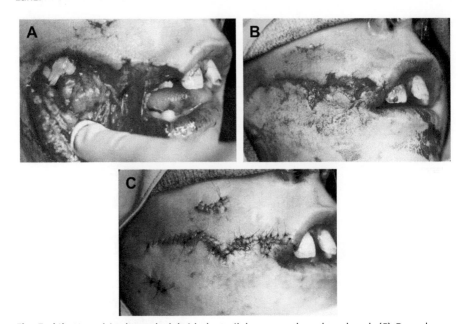

Fig. 7. (*A*) Wound is cleaned, debrided, sterilely prepped, and explored. (*B*) Deep layers, muscle, and subcutaneous tissue are closed to approximate skin, give strength, and eliminate dead space. (*C*) Skin is ultimately easily closed, under much less tension.

edge that is depressed, and more superficial on the higher wound edge. In this manner the edges are leveled. Attempts can be made to make the wound edges perpendicular with the skin surface because this results in a smoother, less noticeable scar. Steri-Strips or butterfly bandages with Mastisol can be placed over sutured or glued lacerations to reinforce the closure and increase its tensile strength. This method is particularly useful if the athlete is returning to play. In some deep lacerations a large reinforcing suture or 2 using a larger-caliber nonresorbable suture like 3-0 or 2-0 silk or nylon can be placed circumferentially wide with deep bites and parallel to the skin closure to reinforce it for athletes returning to play. These reinforcing sutures are temporary and are removed after play. Freshly sutured lacerations are dressed with antibiotic ointment and covered if necessary but can be left uncovered. Cicatrix formation is discouraged and prevented with periodic cleansing with cotton gauze and peroxide and redressed with antibiotic ointment. Skin sutures are generally removed in the face at 5 to 6 days to prevent so-called railroad-track epithelialization of the suture tract. Steri-Strips and Mastisol are recommended for an additional 3 to 5 days until the wound's tensile strength is adequate to resist widening of the scar. Scalp sutures can be left longer; 10 to 14 days if necessary. Deep lacerations of the eyelid, ear, or nose present different challenges because of the tarsal plate or cartilage. Closure of lacerations to these areas is described more thoroughly earlier in this article.

Regarding injuries to collateral soft tissue structures, such as salivary ducts or terminal branches of the facial nerve, injures to these structures are rare. If salivary or lacrimal duct disruption is suspected because of the anatomic location of the wound, the athlete should be evaluated by a specialist because these injuries should be repaired acutely and stented, generally in the operating room while the wound is repaired.

If there are suspected injuries to the terminal branches of cranial nerves in the face (usually the facial nerve, rarely the trigeminal nerve), these athletes should also be evaluated by a specialist. These injuries are rarely repaired acutely, and the laceration must be extensive to involve them. Prompt specialty referral is the best course if any question of injury exists. Complex, deep, or contaminated lacerations or wounds in close proximity to the eyes may be treated with antibiotics. The drug of choice is cephalexin used with clindamycin for allergic patients.

INTRAORAL LACERATIONS

Sports-related intraoral lacerations are common and generally the result of blunt trauma. The injury results from pressure contact of the mucosa of the lips, cheeks, or tongue with the teeth, dental appliances or braces, or even with mouth guards. Traumatic tooth bite injuries to the cheeks and tongue, especially from mandibular trauma, are common too. Isolated intraoral trauma from a direct external cause is rare but may also occur. As in the case of extraoral laceration, hemostasis is of primary concern and can generally be achieved best with direct pressure. Local anesthetics with vasoconstrictors (2% lidocaine, 1:100,000 epinephrine) can be useful, and electrocautery and well-placed sutures can assist with stubborn, persistent bleeding. Hand-held battery-powered electrocautery units can be useful for this purpose.

Wounds are inspected particularly for foreign bodies, and for associated hard tissue or vital structure injuries. In the case of extensive painful wounds, local anesthesia can sometimes be administered first, to help with bleeding and to allow thorough inspection and debridement. Ultimately the anesthesia persists to allow repair (**Fig. 8**).

Superficial intraoral mucosal lacerations are generally best closed with a 3-0 or 4-0 resorbable suture, like chromic gut or polyglycolic acid (Vicryl). In elite athletes, Vicryl is preferred because of its strength, its resistance to knot failure, and its slower resorption. Vicryl Rapide, a quicker resorbing Vicryl but still longer lasting than chromic, is a good substitute. In general, cutting needles like P3 or PS2 are used, but tapered needles (RB-1) can be used for thin, nonkeratinized mucosa. For tongue lacerations, 3-0 Vicryl or silk with larger bites is preferred because of the muscular, active nature of the tongue and the need for stronger suture, particularly on the dorsum and lateral borders. Lacerations of the ventral tongue can be closed like mucosa. The vermillion lip mucosa on the extraoral side of the wet-dry line can be closed like the skin of the lip, with 5-0 nylon or proline. Closure of lacerations in the floor of the mouth or cheek mucosa can be complicated by the position of the salivary ducts. The parotid duct is deep in the cheek and not usually involved in intraoral lacerations. However, the submandibular ducts are superficial in the floor of the mouth and care must be taken not to accidentally ligate the ducts during suturing. Ducts can be tested easily for patency and lack of disruption by milking the ducts and looking for new secretions at the duct orifice.

For the parotid, this means milking the gland from the ear lobe forward and looking for new drops of saliva at the orifice in the cheek mucosa opposite the upper second

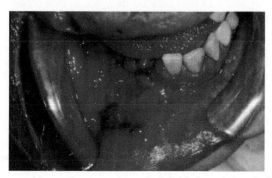

Fig. 8. Intraoral mucosal lacerations are cleaned, debrided, and closed either with chromic gut or polyglycolic acid suture (Vicryl).

molar. For the submandibular ducts, the glands can be milked with pressure over the glands just under the midmandible and looking for new saliva at the orifice in the anterior floor of the mouth under the tongue just behind the lower front teeth. Lack of salivary secretion is cause for further evaluation.

Deeper intraoral lacerations and those with more heavy and persistent bleeding require layered closure. Deeper layers are closed similarly to skin lacerations, with interrupted 3-0 or 4-0 chromic or 4-0 Vicryl or P3 or PS2 cutting needles. The submucosa is closed in an interrupted fashion with 4-0 chromic or P3 or PS2 needles. The mucosa is closed as previously described. Inverting resorbable sutures can be used to close the mucosa to bury knots for patient comfort. With deeper lacerations, sterile prep with povidone iodine solution (Betadine) is vital to reducing infection. Again, for same-day return to play, temporary circumferential reinforcing sutures may be placed and removed at the end of the contest. Additional protective face gear is absolutely indicated to protect the repair, for as long as necessary. Complex, deep, or severely contaminated lacerations may be treated with antibiotics. Penicillin or amoxicillin are the drugs of choice, with clindamycin, or Z pack for patients allergic to penicillin.

THROUGH-AND-THROUGH FACIAL LACERATIONS

Through-and-through lacerations are lacerations of the skin of the face with an intraoral component that directly communicates. They are generally higher-impact injuries from blunt or sharp external trauma, with the intraoral component often associated with secondary tooth trauma. By definition, they transect all layers of the skin and mucosa of the mouth and face and may have increased bleeding (**Fig. 9**).

Initial management of these injuries is the same but additional care must be taken during debridement to totally cleanse the wound through and through. Anesthesia is achieved with a combination of infiltration and blocks, generally with 2% lidocaine 1:100,000 epinephrine. More prolonged anesthesia can be achieved with 0.5% bupivacaine 1:200,000 epinephrine. Intraoral and extraoral nerve block techniques are invaluable for these injuries, particularly the inferior alveolar dental block. The inferior alveolar block together with the simple long buccal nerve block anesthetizes the ipsilateral lip, chin, tongue, mandibular teeth, and lower labial and buccal mucosa for 2 hours with xylocaine and 6 to 8 hours with bupivacaine. The wound is thoroughly prepped sterilely and closure is initiated intraorally. The mucosal component is closed in a watertight fashion with appropriate suture. Then from the outside the wound is reprepped in a sterile fashion and the rest of the closure is done with sterile draping and in a similar fashion to the layered closure for deep facial lacerations (**Fig. 10**).

Through-and-through lacerations are dressed and protected in the same fashion as other lacerations but return to play may be delayed. In elite athletes, depending on severity and situation, return may be immediate with added protection if possible (eg, cage or full-face shield in hockey). For most athletes, time out is usually 1 week. Antibiotics are recommended in all through-through lacerations and the drug of choice is penicillin VK 500 mg every 6 hours for 5 days or amoxicillin 500 mg every 8 hours for 5 days. Clindamycin 300 mg every 8 hours for 5 days is recommended for patients allergic to penicillin.[5,6]

PUNCTURE OR IMPALING WOUNDS

Because of the nature of some athletic activities and equipment, puncture or impaling injuries, although rare, are possible. In puncture wounds, generally the skin laceration length is smaller than the depth. These injuries are therefore innocuous looking but, because of their increased potential for infection, must be cared for meticulously.

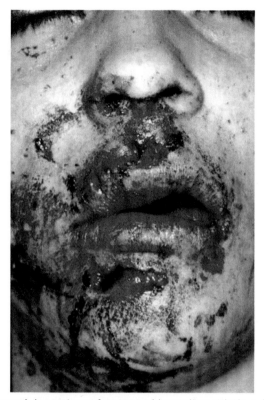

Fig. 9. Through-through lacerations of upper and lower lips with dental injuries.

Hallmarks of therapy are aggressive cleansing and debridement, exploration with attention to possible deep structure damage, layered closure as indicated, and appropriate use of antibiotics.

Impaling injuries are exceedingly rare but can occur. Possible mechanisms are splintered fragments of wood, graphite, or metal from sticks or bats, and collision or falls onto fencing or equipment. In general, impaled objects should be removed only after appropriate imaging and in a controlled setting; namely the clinic or emergency room. Secondary damage is always a concern and bleeding that is obtunded by the object can be brisk when the object is removed. If the impaling object is fixed and cannot be removed safely on site, the object may need to be sectioned so that the athlete may be transported. However, these incidents are rare.

COMPLICATIONS

Complications usually involve infection, scar formation, compromise of function, and (rarely) missed injury. Infection is addressed with debridement and incision and drainage as needed, and addition or substitution of appropriate antibiotics. Scar revision, if necessary, should generally be done after the scar is mature and preferably in the off season. Hypertrophic scar or keloid can be addressed with steroid injections or careful scar revision or dermabrasion in conjunction with steroid injection. Pigmented scars from abrasions that do not improve with time can be treated with bleaching agents or with formal revision.

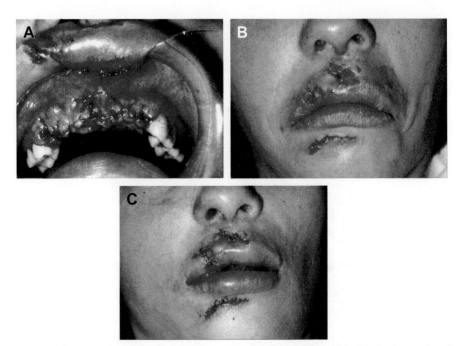

Fig. 10. (*A*) Intraoral mucosa is closed first in watertight fashion. (*B*) Skin is cleansed and prepped. (*C*) Skin closure.

Compromise of function needs to be investigated for cause and treated accordingly. However, functional problems from soft tissue injuries to the face are rare, and generally related to scar tissue. Problems generally improve when the scar is addressed.

In addition, late missed injuries are uncommon, particularly when the injured athlete is evaluated acutely using these established guidelines. In the event of occult or late missed injury, evaluation and treatment by appropriate specialists is key to optimizing return of function.[7]

REFERENCES

1. American College of Surgeons. Advanced trauma life support. Chicago: ACS; 2012.
2. ADA Council on Access, Prevention, and Inter-professional Relations, ADA Council on Scientific Affairs. Using mouthguard to reduce the incidence and severity of sports related injuries. J Am Dent Assoc 2006;137(12):1712–20.
3. Rowe NL, Killey HC. Fractures of the facial skeleton. 2nd edition. Edinburgh (United Kingdom): Livingstone; 1968.
4. Beam JW. Tissue adhesives for simple traumatic lacerations. J Athl Train 2008; 43(2):222–4.
5. Curtin JW. Basic Plastic Surgical Techniques in Repair of Facial Lacerations. Sur Clin of North America 1973;53(1):33–46.
6. Kaufman BR, Heckler FR. Sports-related facial injuries. Clin Sports Med 1997; 16(3):543–62.
7. Roccia F, Diaspro A, Nasi A, et al. Management of sports-related maxillofacial injuries. J Craniofac Surg 2008;19(2):377–82.

Eye and Orbital Injuries in Sports

Jonathan A. Micieli, MD, CM[a], Michael Easterbrook, MD, FRCSC[b],*

KEYWORDS

• Eye injuries • Sports • Globe rupture • Eye protection

KEY POINTS

• Eye protection prevents serious eye injuries in sports.
• Certain findings on history or physical examination warrant urgent referral to an ophthalmologist.
• Irreversible blindness may occur after sports-related trauma.

Although sports-related eye injuries are completely preventable they continue to occur, with serious consequences. Prevention is the most effective way to eliminate the significant morbidity and costs associated with sports-related eye injuries.[1,2] However, for various reasons, including noncompliance with regulations, the lack of enforcement, or suboptimal legislation, these injuries continue to occur regularly.[3–5] Eye trauma has significant consequences not only to the individual but also to society. There is a tremendous cost to care for and treat individuals who have sustained a sports-related injury and many experience permanent vision loss, which has profound effects on their lives.[6] This article discusses the mechanisms, classification, and specific sports-related injuries that may occur to the eye and orbit. It ends with a brief discussion on eye protection and ocular motor function in concussion.

MECHANISM OF INJURY

Trauma to the eye may occur by blunt, penetrating, or perforating mechanisms. Blunt injuries refer to contusions or forces that strike an intact globe. Penetrating injuries occur when there is a single laceration to the eye causing an open globe, and perforating injuries occur when 2 full-thickness lacerations (entrance and exit) are present and are usually caused by a sharp object or missile.

Disclosure: The authors have no conflicts of interest to disclose.
^a Department of Ophthalmology and Vision Sciences, University of Toronto, 340 College Street, Suite 400, Toronto, Ontario M5T 2S8, Canada; ^b Department of Ophthalmology and Vision Sciences, University of Toronto, Suite 310, 790 Bay Street, Toronto, Ontario M5G 1N8, Canada
* Corresponding author.
E-mail address: michael.easterbrook@sympatico.ca

Clin Sports Med 36 (2017) 299–314
http://dx.doi.org/10.1016/j.csm.2016.11.006
sportsmed.theclinics.com

The severity of an eye injury is correlated with the total impact force, the force onset rate, and the kinetic energy of an object.[7] Experimental studies performed on human, monkey, and porcine eyes show that, after impact, the sclera expands equatorially, producing corneoscleral stress that can cause rupture of the eye.[8,9] Computational models of the eye have been used to simulate a variety of impacts and analyze injury potential. An example of this is the Virginia Tech–Wake Forest University (VT-WFU) eye model, which is a finite element model that has been validated to predict globe rupture for blunt eye impacts.[10] This model has shown that stresses in the corneoscleral shell exceeding 23 MPa and local dynamic pressures exceeding 2.1 MPa result in globe rupture.[10] Other studies have shown that spherical projectiles (baseballs, BB pellets, paintballs, airsoft pellets) result in higher stresses and pressures in the eye compared with cylindrical projectiles (blunt impactor, aluminum, foam) and that peak stresses are located at the apex of the cornea, the limbus, or the equator of the globe.[11] Models such as this can be used as predictive aids to reduce the burden and better understand the mechanisms of eye injury.

CLASSIFICATION OF INJURIES

Sports-related eye injuries can be classified using the Birmingham Eye Trauma Terminology (**Fig. 1**).[12] This classification system uses the entire globe as the tissue of reference and has been endorsed by various societies of ocular trauma. In this system, an eye injury is first classified as either a closed globe injury or an open globe injury. Closed globe injuries can be further subdivided as either contusions (meaning there is no scleral or corneal wound) or lamellar lacerations (partial-thickness wounds of the eye wall). Open globe injuries are further divided into ruptures (full-thickness wound caused by blunt object) or lacerations (full-thickness wound of the eye wall caused by a sharp object). Lacerations can be penetrating, perforating, or involve an intraocular foreign body, which is a retained foreign body causing an entrance laceration.

ANATOMY OF THE EYE AND ORBIT

The eye or globe is not a true sphere. The radius of curvature of the cornea (8 mm) is smaller than that of the sclera (12 mm), giving it the shape of an oblate spheroid.[13] The anteroposterior diameter of the globe is usually between 23 and 25 mm, with myopes (near-sighted individuals) generally having longer eyes than hyperopes (far-sighted individuals). The eye is divided into 3 main compartments: the anterior chamber, the

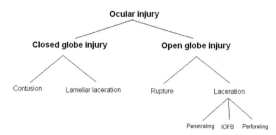

Fig. 1. Classification of sports-related eye injuries. IOFB, intraocular foreign body. (*Courtesy of* Birmingham Eye Trauma Terminology; *adapted from* Kuhn F, Morris R, Witherspoon CD, et al. A standardized classification of ocular trauma. Graefes Arch Clin Exp Ophthalmol 1996;234(6):399–403; with permission.)

posterior chamber, and the vitreous cavity. The anterior chamber refers to the space between the front surface of the eye (cornea) and the iris, whereas the posterior chamber refers to the space between the posterior portion of the iris and the anterior vitreous face. The vitreous cavity occupies that largest volume of the eye (5–6 mL).

There are some important anatomic features of the eye relevant to sports-related injuries that should be highlighted. The sclera, which is the white, outer layer of the eye, is thinnest (0.3 mm) just posterior to the insertion of the rectus muscles and therefore globe rupture is most likely to occur at this location, at the equator of the globe, and at the corneal limbus (junction of the cornea and sclera). The limbus serves as a source of stem cells whose division serves to maintain the corneal epithelium and replace lost cells from corneal abrasions.[14] The aqueous humor is the fluid that fills the anterior chamber and is made by the ciliary body and circulates in this space until it drains in the trabecular meshwork, which is located at the junction of the iris and the cornea. Contusions to the eye may result in the dispersion of blood (hyphema) or pigment that may decrease the outflow at the trabecular meshwork and result in an increased intraocular pressure.

The eye lies within the orbit, which has a volume of about 30 cm^3.[13] Each orbit is composed of 7 different bones that form a roof, floor, and medial and lateral wall. The lateral orbital wall is the thickest and strongest of the walls and is formed from 2 bones: the zygomatic and greater wing of the sphenoid. The medial orbital wall is the thinnest because it is composed of the lamina papyracea, a thin covering of the ethmoidal sinuses. The shortest of the orbital walls is the orbital floor, which does not extend to the orbital apex, but instead ends at the pterygopalatine fossa. The infraorbital canal located 4 mm below the inferior orbital margin transmits the infraorbital nerve, which is a branch of V_2 (maxillary division of the trigeminal nerve). Sports-related trauma to the orbit may result in injury or fracture to the bones, nerve, or vascular supply located within this space.

FIRST RESPONSE TO A POTENTIAL EYE INJURY

Evaluation of an athlete who sustained a potential eye injury on the sidelines begins with reviewing the mechanism of injury. This review may include interviewing the patient, spectators, or teammates, or reviewing film footage at a later date. A review of the symptoms the athlete has experienced is critical to developing a differential diagnosis and deciding on the need for and timing of referral to an ophthalmologist. It is also important to note whether the athlete was wearing glasses or contact lenses because rigid contact lenses have the potential to cause corneal abrasions or lacerations given their design with sharp edges.

Symptoms that warrant referral to an ophthalmologist are summarized in **Table 1**. A physical examination on the sidelines should begin with testing visual acuity 1 eye at a time. An examination of the pupils with a penlight and assessment of extraocular movements should follow. Assessment of the adnexa and the globe should then be performed with a penlight and using fluorescein eye drops with a cobalt blue light to assess the surface of the cornea if necessary. It is also important to have cotton swabs and eye-irrigating fluids available in case an ocular foreign body is detected. Some physical examination signs that warrant urgent referral to an ophthalmologist are summarized in **Table 2**.

OPEN GLOBE INJURIES

If an open globe injury is suspected, it requires urgent attention by the medical staff on a sports team and an urgent referral to an ophthalmologist. These injuries may occur

Table 1
Ocular symptoms in athletes that warrant an urgent referral to an ophthalmologist

Symptom	Potential Problem
1. Loss of vision	Various (nonspecific complaint)
2. Diplopia (double vision)	Extraocular muscle entrapment in orbital fracture Cranial nerve injury
3. Photophobia	Anterior chamber inflammation (traumatic iritis, microhyphema)
4. Flashes ± floaters	Vitreous detachment Retinal tear
5. Visual field defect	Retinal detachment
6. Ocular pain with foreign-body sensation	Corneal abrasion
7. Ocular pain with nausea/vomiting	Increased intraocular pressure

with severe blunt injuries or by penetrating or perforating mechanisms. Athletes with open globe injuries complain of severe pain and reduced vision. Physical examination may reveal dramatic findings, such as a deformed globe or extrusion of intraocular contents, or more subtle findings, such as an irregular pupil or a small corneal laceration (**Fig. 2**). If an open globe injury is suspected, no pressure should be placed on the eye and a shield should be placed to prevent any further accidental contact with the eye. An urgent evaluation is then required by an ophthalmologist.

Open globe injuries require urgent surgical repair to ensure that the globe is closed. Depending on the mechanism of injury, a computed tomography (CT) scan of the orbits may be required to ensure that there is no intraocular foreign body. An open globe with an intraocular foreign body requires a different surgical approach. Timely closure of the open wound is required in the operating room to reduce the risk of infection and permanent loss of vision. Previous studies have shown that factors associated with a poor prognosis are younger age, poor initial visual acuity, and posterior segment involvement.[15] After surgical intervention, patients must be closely monitored because

Table 2
Physical examination findings in athletes that warrant an urgent referral to an ophthalmologist

Examination Finding	Potential Problem
1. Unequal visual acuity in one eye compared with the other	Various (nonspecific problem)
2. Unequal pupils	Traumatic mydriasis Anterior chamber inflammation
3. Restricted extraocular movements	Extraocular muscle entrapment in orbital fracture Cranial nerve injury
4. Photophobia with penlight examination	Anterior chamber inflammation (traumatic iritis, microhyphema)
5. Iris not visualized in detail	Anterior chamber inflammation (traumatic iritis, microhyphema) Corneal injury Increased intraocular pressure

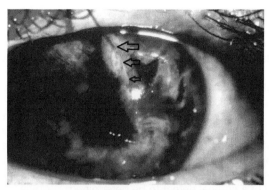

Fig. 2. External view of the eye revealing a corneal laceration. Iris can be seen in the corneal wounds (*arrows*). This patient requires urgent surgical management to close the corneal wound.

they may develop other ocular conditions, such as retinal detachment or glaucoma, in the future.

CLOSED GLOBE INJURIES

Nonpenetrating trauma can result in a wide variety of tissue damage to the cornea, iris, lens, vitreous, choroid, and retina. The expansion of the eyeball perpendicular to the direction of impact has been proposed to be responsible for the injuries that occur from blunt trauma.[1] The large stresses cause a significant amount of distortion in the anatomy of the eye and result in tearing of structures such as the cornea, pupillary sphincter, ciliary body, trabecular meshwork, lens zonules, and peripheral retina. These injuries are discussed in further detail later.

Corneal and Conjunctival Injuries

The cornea is a transparent, avascular tissue that measures approximately 11 to 12 mm in horizontal diameter and provides most of the refractive power of the eye. The cornea has one of the highest densities of nerve endings in the body, receiving its innervation from the ophthalmic branch of the trigeminal nerve.[16] The cornea is composed of 5 major layers from the superficial epithelium, Bowman layer, stroma, Descemet membrane, and the endothelium.[17] The aqueous humor provides the glucose and the tear film provides the oxygen for the cornea's nutritional needs. The conjunctiva is a thin, transparent mucous membrane that covers the sclera and inner linings of the eyelid. The conjunctiva may become red after a direct injury or as a secondary reaction to an injury or disease process elsewhere in the eye.

Corneal abrasion

Among the most frequent sports-related injuries is the corneal abrasion, which is a defect of the superficial epithelium that almost always occurs secondary to trauma in sports-related settings. Corneal abrasions account for more than 10% of the ocular injuries in the National Basketball Association and more than 20% of soccer ball–related injuries in young amateur athletes.[18,19] Abrasions are also frequently seen in wrestling, martial arts, boxing, and rugby and occur when either a finger or ball comes into contact with the cornea.[20] Once the corneal epithelium is traumatically removed, immediate pain, foreign-body sensation, and tearing may be experienced by the athlete. Given the intense and immediate pain, corneal abrasions require prompt attention to assess the eye and rule out any associated injuries.

External examination of the cornea can be performed with a penlight and should begin with an assessment of the position and action of the eyelids and overall assessment of the globe. Because a corneal abrasion is a superficial injury, the pain from this injury resolves with an application of topical anesthetic such as proparacaine hydrochloride or tetracaine. Topical fluorescein is a nontoxic, water-soluble dye that makes corneal abrasions more evident because it detects disruption of intercellular junctions and stains areas of absent epithelium fluorescent green in the presence of cobalt blue light (**Fig. 3**).[21] Examination of the cornea can be performed in greater detail with slit-lamp biomicroscopy, but is not usually available on the sidelines. This tool allows an assessment of the cornea in greater detail and provides a cross-sectional view that enables the depth of a corneal defect to be determined.

Corneal abrasions are usually managed with topical antibiotics (drops or ointment) to prevent infection.[21,22] Topical nonsteroidal antiinflammatory agents (ketorolac tromethamine [Acular], nepafenac [Nevanac], or diclofenac sodium [Voltaren]) may also be used for the first 24 to 48 hours for pain relief in selected patients; however, they should be used with caution because they can cause local toxicity. Therapeutic contact lenses and patching may also be used in larger abrasions with significant pain, but should be used in conjunction with an ophthalmologist.

Corneal injuries after refractive surgery

Refractive surgery, including radial keratotomy (RK) and laser in situ keratomileusis (LASIK), have been used for the treatment of myopia (nearsightedness) and hyperopia (farsightedness). RK involves making deep radial corneal incisions with a diamond knife to flatten the central cornea for mild to moderate myopia.[23] However, this procedure is now considered obsolete, primarily because of the continuing long-term instability of the procedure.[23] RK also weakens the cornea to a great extent. An eye that has had RK ruptures through the RK incisions with about half the force required to rupture an unincised eye.[24] Previous studies have shown that RK incisions become the weakest point in the eye, leading to an increased risk of globe rupture after blunt trauma.[25] Consequently, protective polycarbonate eyewear is of the utmost importance in patients who have undergone RK.

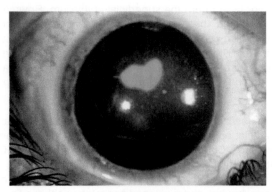

Fig. 3. External view of the eye revealing a corneal abrasion highlighted with topical fluorescein. The fluorescein dye stains the de-epithelialized area when examined with cobalt blue light.

The LASIK procedure is performed with a microkeratome or femtosecond laser to create a corneal flap approximately 15% to 35% of the corneal thickness.[26] After the flap is lifted, an excimer laser is used to ablate the remaining corneal bed in the visual axis to correct myopia, hyperopia, or astigmatism. Traumatic dislocation of the LASIK flap has been reported many months or even years following surgery.[27] Sports-related traumatic dislocations and amputations of the LASIK flap may also occur and requires immediate attention by an ophthalmologist.[27,28] Flap loss is a serious complication because severe and unpredictable refractive error may occur, emphasizing the importance of using polycarbonate protective eyewear in these athletes.

Subconjunctival hemorrhage

Subconjunctival hemorrhage is a common condition that occurs when a blood vessel ruptures and blood accumulates in the subconjunctival space. Common causes include trauma, hypertension, anticoagulant therapy, and increased venous pressure (Valsalva, coughing, vomiting).[29] Sports-related blunt trauma is a common cause of subconjunctival hemorrhage and may occur in almost all settings.[30] This condition does not cause pain or vision changes and is mainly a cosmetic issue. It manifests as diffuse areas of redness that contrasts sharply with the underlying adjacent white sclera (**Fig. 4**). No treatment is necessary because the blood resorbs spontaneously and there are no sequelae. Small hemorrhages usually take 2 to 3 days to resolve, whereas large hemorrhages may take up to 2 weeks. However, large amounts of 360° of subconjunctival hemorrhage may be harbingers of a more severe underlying penetrating injury and must be referred urgently to an ophthalmologist if this is suspected.

Anterior and Posterior Segment Injuries

Important anatomic structures in the anterior segment (located between the cornea and iris) and posterior segment (located between the lens and anterior vitreous face) are the iris, lens, and trabecular meshwork. The iris is composed of the blood vessels, connective tissue, melanocytes, and pigment cells that are responsible for its distinctive color. The mobility of the iris allows the pupil to change size and respond to changes in light. The lens is an important biconvex structure that contributes focusing power to the eye. It is held in place by a system of zonular fibers that are made of fibrillin fibers that may weaken or rupture because of trauma.

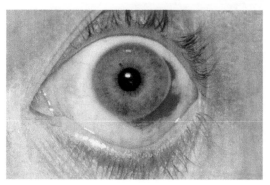

Fig. 4. Subconjunctival hemorrhage seen in the temporal part of the eye from blunt trauma. The hemorrhage appears dark red in contrast with the adjacent white sclera.

Traumatic hyphema

A traumatic hyphema is the entry of blood in the anterior chamber and may be seen with a penlight as layering of blood at the inferior part of the cornea. Trauma causes scleral expansion in the equatorial zone and disruption of the major iris arterial circle and arterial branches of the ciliary body, which results in blood in the anterior chamber. Hyphemas are common injuries in sports in both children and adults and occur with blunt trauma.[31,32] They have been reported to occur more often in male participants (approximately 3:1) and in sports such as baseball, basketball, soccer, racquet sports, and combat.[31,33,34] A hyphema requires urgent referral to an ophthalmologist for evaluation.

Traumatic hyphemas may be fairly asymptomatic or present with significant pain and decreased vision. The pain may be a result of associated corneal injuries or secondary to increased intraocular pressure (IOP), which occurs because of obstruction of the trabecular meshwork (aqueous drainage pathway) by red blood cells, fibrin, or other debris.[34,35] Uncontrolled IOP can lead to irreversible damage to the optic nerve and therefore must be monitored by an ophthalmologist during the course of the condition. Treatment may require topical medications or even surgery if the IOP cannot be controlled medically.[35] Another concern with hyphemas is the possibility of rebleeding, which has been reported to occur in about 18% of patients between 3 and 5 days after the injury.[36] Rebleeding is of particular concern in patients with sickle-cell disease who have been found to have enhanced fibrinolysis.[37]

Traumatic cataract

Blunt injury to the eye may also result in a cataract because of disruption of the organized lens proteins. It may involve the entire lens or be segmental (**Fig. 5**). A common pattern after trauma is a petalloid or rosette-shaped cataract in which each petal is separated by a linear suture line in the lens.[38] A traumatic cataract may be difficult to visualize in the absence of pupil dilatation because the iris covers most of the lens, especially in bright conditions. In a dark room or with dilatation, a cataract appears as a white to brown discoloration of the lens that precludes a detailed image of the fundus. In the setting of a traumatic cataract, there is a high incidence of disruption of the zonular fibers, which hold the lens in position.[39] This condition may result in lens subluxation or dislocation (**Fig. 6**). Any patients with reduced vision, including findings that suggest a traumatic cataract, require referral to an ophthalmologist.

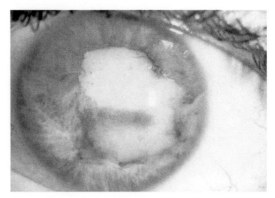

Fig. 5. Traumatic cataract that developed several weeks after blunt trauma. There is also associated iris injury.

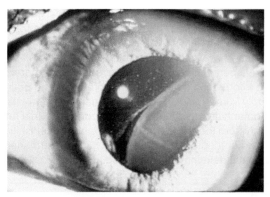

Fig. 6. Lens dislocation after blunt trauma. The edge of the lens can be seen in the center of the pupil.

Traumatic cataract may cause mild to significant loss of vision. When there is significant vision loss that interferes with the patient's quality of life, cataract surgery is indicated. This surgery involves making microincisions in the cornea, removal of the lens with high-energy ultrasonography, and insertion of an artificial intraocular lens. Because the artificial lens does not have the same accommodative ability of the natural crystalline lens, spectacle correction is usually necessary to allow for near vision.[40] If there is significant loss or disruption of the lens zonules, the intraocular lens will not center in the normal lens capsule, but may need to be fixated to the sclera or placed in the anterior chamber.[39]

Vitreous Cavity Injuries

The vitreous occupies approximately 80% of the volume of the eye. It is a clear matrix composed mainly of water and hyaluronic acid. The vitreous is firmly attached to the vitreous base (an area in the peripheral retina), retinal vessels, macula, and optic nerve. With increasing age, pockets of liquefaction develop and the vitreous gel eventually starts to shrink, putting parts of the retina under traction.[41] This traction can lead to spontaneous breaks in the retina, which can be visualized as horseshoe tears or operculated holes in the fundus (**Fig. 7**). These breaks permit the movement of

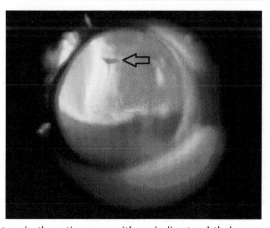

Fig. 7. Horseshoe tear in the retina seen with an indirect ophthalmoscope (*arrow*).

liquefied vitreous into the subretinal space, which can cause the retina to detach **(Fig. 8)**.[41] Blunt trauma in sports may cause similar changes in the vitreous and subsequent traction on the retina. If this force is severe enough it may result in a vitreous hemorrhage, retinal tear, or retinal detachment.

The retina is the transparent film of the eye that contains photoreceptors that translate light stimuli into information that can be interpreted by the brain.[42] The retina receives its blood supply from 2 major sources: the inner half of the retina from the retinal circulation and the outer half from the choroidal circulation.[43] In a retinal detachment, the outer blood supply from the choroid is no longer able to nourish the retina, resulting in damage to the photoreceptors. This damage can be permanent if enough time passes before the retinal detachment is repaired.

Retinal detachment

In sports settings, retinal detachments may occur in isolation or in conjunction with other ocular or orbital injuries. The most common symptom elicited by patients with a retinal detachment are a history of flashes and floaters.[44] Flashes represent the retinal response to traction from the vitreous gel and floaters represent mobile condensations in the vitreous gel that project a dark shadow onto the retina. When the retina starts to detach, the patient notices a defect corresponding with the area of detached retina. Because the superior retina interprets the inferior visual field and vice versa, a superior retinal detachment manifests as an inferior visual field defect. If left untreated, this visual field progresses to involve the central vision and the entire visual field. Therefore, patients with these symptoms require urgent evaluation and treatment by an ophthalmologist.

The prognosis for retinal detachment is improved when the detached retina is localized and does not involve the macula, or central retina. These so-called macula-on detachments are considered urgent and require immediate attention to prevent further retinal involvement. When a larger part of the retina is detached and involves the macula, a macula-off detachment, the treatment is less urgent. Similar outcomes have been reported for macula-off detachments with immediate treatment and treatment within 1-week of symptom onset.[45,46] Treatment options include office-based procedures, such as pneumatic retinopexy, which involves the injection of an intraocular gas bubble and laser around the retinal break. Other surgical options include pars plana vitrectomy and scleral buckling.[45]

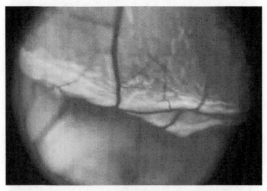

Fig. 8. Retinal detachment seen with an indirect ophthalmoscope. The elevated retina can be seen with the retinal vessels in the superior part of the image.

Vitreous hemorrhage
Blunt ocular trauma may cause vitreous traction that results in a rupture of a retinal blood vessel and hemorrhage into the vitreous. Patients report diffuse blurry vision that may have a red-tinged appearance. Physical examination may reveal the absence of a red reflex with the direct ophthalmoscope because the blood obscures visualization of the fundus. Patients require urgent referral to an ophthalmologist to rule out a concomitant retinal detachment, which can be detected by ultrasonography. When there is no retinal detachment, treatment involves conservative measures, including avoiding vigorous activity and sleeping with the head of the bed elevated, which allows the hemorrhage to clear. Close observation is required because there is a high incidence of retinal breaks in this population, which may lead to a retinal detachment in the future.[47]

Orbital injuries
Injuries to the orbit may occur in conjunction with ocular injuries or may be isolated. One of the most frequent facial injuries in sports is orbital bone fracture, which is leading cause of injury from blunt trauma in fighting in hockey, boxing, and martial arts.[48] Patients who sustain an orbital bone fracture may present with symptoms that vary from mild pain at the site of injury to reduced vision, severe pain, and diplopia. The diplopia can be secondary to extraocular muscle injury, muscle entrapment within a fracture, or orbital hemorrhage. When an orbital bone fracture is suspected, a CT scan of the orbits is the test of choice to confirm the diagnosis because the orbital bones are well visualized. It is always important to rule out a concomitant globe injury, especially when there is significant periorbital edema and the eye cannot be easily visualized. Surgical repair of the fracture is indicated if there is diplopia when looking straight ahead or in the reading position, significant enophthalmos (sunken eye), or a very large fracture.

Other injuries in the orbit can involve injuries to the extraocular muscles from blunt trauma, such as hematomas. The cranial nerves may be injured in the orbit or as they enter through the superior orbital fissure in the setting of orbital bone fracture. Abnormalities in extraocular movements or the position of the globe, such as enophthalmos or exophthalmos, warrant urgent consultation with an ophthalmologist.

EYE PROTECTION

The occurrence of the serious eye injuries discussed earlier can be completely prevented with the use of proper protection. Sport-specific issues related to eye protection are discussed later.

Racquet Sports

Racquet sports, such as squash, badminton, and racquet ball, have a high risk of eye injuries because of the small ball and high velocity at which the game is played.[49] Contrary to popular belief, experienced players are at high risk of eye injuries.[50,51] In 1983, the United States Squash Racquets Association required all participants in national championships to wear eye protection meeting American Society Testing and Materials (ASTM) standard F803.[1] The ASTM F803 is a rigorous standard used in sports and testing requires that no eye contact be made by a squash or racquetball traveling at speeds of 90 mph when hitting the eye protectors from the front or side.[52] The material of these glasses is polycarbonate, which is a highly shatter-resistant material with approximately 150 times the strength of the material in conventional glasses.[53] There have been no reports of significant ocular injury when ASTM eye guards are worn in squash or racquetball.

Hockey

Professional and amateur sports associations have varying legislation with regard to the use of eye protection in hockey. The National Collegiate Athletic Association (NCAA) requires all players to wear full-face cages and there has been no significant eye injury reported in this setting. The National Hockey League in June 2013 mandated that all nonrookie players must wear half-visors, and the number of eye and orbital injuries has continued to decline as more players use visors.[48,54,55] Studies have found that younger players are using half-visors at a faster pace than would be expected from mandatory legislation.[56]

Despite increased use of half-visors in professional and junior hockey leagues, serious eye injuries continue to occur.[48] One reason for this is that the visors are not being worn in the proper position (angled upward with too much space between the nose and visor). Even when worn in the proper position (with not more than 1 finger able to fit between the visor and nose), half-visors are not adequate to prevent all injuries[57] because the force of a high stick, body check, or deflected puck is usually sufficient to cause a shift in the helmet and leave the upper face exposed. In addition, fighting, which is the third leading cause of eye and orbital injuries in hockey, usually takes place without the use of helmets, leaving the eyes exposed to a punch.[48] A new trend of longer, three-quarter visors is starting to gain popularity in professional hockey leagues and may contribute to the further prevention of eye injuries in hockey.[56] Further collaboration between amateur and professional hockey leagues and ophthalmologists is required to study the eye injuries that continue to occur and to optimize protective equipment.[55] However, the National Hockey League and the National Hockey League Players Association has not been willing to collaborate with this group of physicians in studying eye injuries.

Lacrosse

Facial protection with cages is mandatory for male lacrosse players at the amateur and professional levels and no significant eye injuries have occurred with this equipment. However, according to the international women's lacrosse rules, eye guards may be worn but are not mandatory for women.[58] Previous studies have shown that the use of protective eyewear was associated with a decrease in eye injuries in women's lacrosse.[59] Recently, United States Lacrosse has introduced new legislation and an eyewear standard, ASTM 3077, that will become mandatory in 2017. Expanding the progress that United States Lacrosse has made in mandating eye protection in this sport is required in other regions and leagues to adequately protect athletes.

Paintball

Although use of ocular protection is mandatory at most paintball sites, most injuries are caused by not following the rules and not using eye protection at all times.[60] Acrylic goggles provide adequate protection provided that they have a tight seal to the face.[61] Ensuring a good fit to the goggles with no space between the skin and frame is important because serious ocular injuries have been reported when the paintball goes underneath the eye protection.[62] Newer facial gear that has full facial protection and goggles that permit a wide field of view can help overcome any visual limitations of traditional goggles.[62]

Other Sports and Considerations for Eye Protection

Significant eye injuries have been reported in baseball and basketball and polycarbonate eye or facial protection is available, although it has not become widely popular.[18]

Other sports, such as soccer, wrestling, rugby, and water polo, do not have accepted standards for eye protection and present a unique challenge because of the difficulty of wearing protection during the games. Any monocular athlete should always wear polycarbonate eye protection in any sport in which there is potential for injury. Extra precaution should be taken in sports like hockey in which it is recommended that polycarbonate eyewear be used underneath a full face shield.[53]

OCULAR MOTOR ASSESSMENT IN CONCUSSION

Concussion is increasingly being recognized as a public health concern and there is a need to develop sensitive tests to detect and evaluate the brain dysfunction that occurs in this condition. More than half of the brain's circuitry is involved in eye movements and vision and this is corroborated by the common visual complaints that are seen in concussed athletes.[63,64] Saccades and smooth pursuit are two types of eye movements that have shown abnormalities with detailed testing in concussed athletes.[65] The former refers to rapidly shifting simultaneous movements of the eyes from one target to another, whereas the latter involves the eyes slowly following an object. Previous studies have also shown that concussed athletes have difficulties with accommodation and increased levels of photophobia.[64]

Testing complex visuospatial tasks in athletes may provide valuable information in determining when an athlete should be removed from play, especially when the athlete does not endorse any concussive symptoms after taking a hit in a game. The King-Devick test is one such sideline test that allows a rapid, reliable, and objective assessment of an athlete.[66] This test requires patients to read numbers with variable spacing as quickly as possible on 3 test cards. Because saccades, attention, and language are required to read these cards quickly, diffuse networks in the brain are being evaluated, including the areas for saccade generation. At the beginning of a season, baseline testing is performed, which serves as a reference to evaluate the same athlete if that athlete experiences an injury. Worsening of the time required to complete the test provides objective evidence to remove the player from play. In a meta-analysis evaluating the ability of the King-Devick test to detect concussions in sports such as hockey, lacrosse, football, basketball, soccer, and boxing, the test was found to have a sensitivity and specificity of 90% and 86%, respectively.[67] On average, baseline times worsened by 4.8 seconds in concussed athletes.

In summary, eye and orbital injuries are significant risks to athletes and can result in permanent blindness. Eye injuries can be classified as open or closed globe injuries and red flags in the history or physical examination should alert the first responder to arrange an urgent ophthalmology consultation. Eye protection is available for most sports and should be worn in accordance with the standards of regional authorities. Protective eyewear should be made from polycarbonate material to ensure the highest levels of safety. Vision and eye movements involve a large proportion of the brain's circuitry and can provide objective evidence of brain dysfunction in athletes suspected of having a concussion.

REFERENCES

1. Vinger P. The eye and sports medicine. In: Tasman W, Jaeger JE, editors. Duane's ophthalmology. Philadelphia: Lippincott Williams & Wilkins; 2007.

2. Bell JA. Eye trauma in sports: a preventable epidemic. JAMA 1981;246:156.

3. Gordon KD. The incidence of eye injuries in Canada. Can J Ophthalmol 2012;47:351–3.

4. Leivo T, Haavisto AK, Sahraravand A. Sports-related eye injuries: the current picture. Acta Ophthalmol 2015;93:224–31.

5. Pollard KA, Xiang H, Smith GA. Pediatric eye injuries treated in US emergency departments, 1990-2009. Clin Pediatr 2012;51:374–81.

6. Vinger PF. Sports eye injuries a preventable disease. Ophthalmology 1981;88:108–13.

7. Berger RE. A model for evaluating the ocular contusion injury potential of propelled objects. J Bioeng 1978;2:345–58.

8. Delori F, Pomerantzeff O, Cox MS. Deformation of the globe under high-speed impact: it relation to contusion injuries. Invest Ophthalmol 1969;8:290–301.

9. Green RP Jr, Peters DR, Shore JW, et al. Force necessary to fracture the orbital floor. Ophthal Plast Reconstr Surg 1990;6:211–7.

10. Stitzel JD, Duma SM, Cormier JM, et al. A nonlinear finite element model of the eye with experimental validation for the prediction of globe rupture. Stapp Car Crash J 2002;46:81–102.

11. Weaver AA, Kennedy EA, Duma SM, et al. Evaluation of different projectiles in matched experimental eye impact simulations. J Biomech Eng 2011;133:031002.

12. Kuhn F, Morris R, Witherspoon CD, et al. A standardized classification of ocular trauma. Graefes Arch Clin Exp Ophthalmol 1996;234:399–403.

13. American Academy of Ophthalmology. Fundamentals and principles of ophthalmology. San Francisco (CA): American Academy of Ophthalmology; 2014-15.

14. Funderburgh JL, Funderburgh ML, Du Y. Stem cells in the limbal stroma. Ocul Surf 2016;14:113–20.

15. Li X, Zarbin MA, Bhagat N. Pediatric open globe injury: a review of the literature. J Emerg Trauma Shock 2015;8:216–23.

16. Millodot M. A review of research on the sensitivity of the cornea. Ophthalmic Physiol Opt 1984;4:305–18.

17. Jalbert I, Stapleton F, Papas E, et al. In vivo confocal microscopy of the human cornea. Br J Ophthalmol 2003;87:225–36.

18. Zagelbaum BM, Starkey C, Hersh PS, et al. The National Basketball Association eye injury study. Arch Ophthalmol 1995;113:749–52.

19. Burke MJ, Sanitato JJ, Vinger PF, et al. Soccerball-induced eye injuries. JAMA 1983;249:2682–5.

20. Orlando RG, Doty JH. Ocular sports trauma: a private practice study. J Am Optom Assoc 1996;67:77–80.

21. Ahmed F, House RJ, Feldman BH. Corneal abrasions and corneal foreign bodies. Prim Care 2015;42:363–75.

22. Wilson SA, Last A. Management of corneal abrasions. Am Fam Physician 2004;70:123–8.

23. Waring GO 3rd, Lynn MJ, McDonnell PJ. Results of the Prospective Evaluation of Radial Keratotomy (PERK) study 10 years after surgery. Arch Ophthalmol 1994;112:1298–308.

24. Larson BC, Kremer FB, Eller AW, et al. Quantitated trauma following radial keratotomy in rabbits. Ophthalmology 1983;90:660–7.

25. Vinger PF, Mieler WF, Oestreicher JH, et al. Ruptured globes following radial and hexagonal keratotomy surgery. Arch Ophthalmol 1996;114:129–34.

26. Wilson SE. Clinical practice. Use of lasers for vision correction of nearsightedness and farsightedness. N Engl J Med 2004;351:470–5.

27. Booth MA, Koch DD. Late laser in situ keratomileusis flap dislocation caused by a thrown football. J Cataract Refract Surg 2003;29:2032–3.

28. Tetz M, Werner L, Muller M, et al. Late traumatic LASIK flap loss during contact sport. J Cataract Refract Surg 2007;33:1332–5.
29. Fukuyama J, Hayasaka S, Yamada K, et al. Causes of subconjunctival hemorrhage. Ophthalmologica 1990;200:63–7.
30. Kent JS, Eidsness RB, Colleaux KM, et al. Indoor soccer-related eye injuries: should eye protection be mandatory? Can J Ophthalmol 2007;42:605–8.
31. DiFiori JP. Sports-related traumatic hyphema. Am Fam Physician 1992;46: 807–13.
32. SooHoo JR, Davies BW, Braverman RS, et al. Pediatric traumatic hyphema: a review of 138 consecutive cases. J AAPOS 2013;17:565–7.
33. Stilger VG, Alt JM, Robinson TW. Traumatic hyphema in an intercollegiate baseball player: a case report. J Athl Train 1999;34:25–8.
34. Johnson D, Schweitzer K, Ten Hove M, et al. Ophthaproblem. Can you identify this condition? Hyphema. Can Fam Physician 2011;57:319, 321–2.
35. Campagna J. Traumatic hyphema: current strategies. Focal Points: Clin Modules Ophthalmologists. San Francisco (CA): American Academy of Ophthalmology; 2007;25:1–14.
36. Rahmani B, Jahadi HR, Rajaeefard A. An analysis of risk for secondary hemorrhage in traumatic hyphema. Ophthalmology 1999;106:380–5.
37. Hagger D, Wolff S, Owen J, et al. Changes in coagulation and fibrinolysis in patients with sickle cell disease compared with healthy black controls. Blood Coagul Fibrinolysis 1995;6:93–9.
38. Ram J, Gupta R. Images in clinical medicine. Petaloid Cataract. N Engl J Med 2016;374:e22.
39. Salehi-Had H, Turalba A. Management of traumatic crystalline lens subluxation and dislocation. Int Ophthalmol Clin 2010;50:167–79.
40. Micieli JA, Arshinoff SA. Cataract surgery. CMAJ 2011;183:1621.
41. Hollands H, Johnson D, Brox AC, et al. Acute-onset floaters and flashes: is this patient at risk for retinal detachment? JAMA 2009;302:2243–9.
42. Grossniklaus HE, Geisert EE, Nickerson JM. Introduction to the retina. Prog Mol Biol Transl Sci 2015;134:383–96.
43. Hosoya K, Tachikawa M. The inner blood-retinal barrier: molecular structure and transport biology. Adv Exp Med Biol 2012;763:85–104.
44. Johnson D, Hollands H. Acute-onset floaters and flashes. CMAJ 2012;184:431.
45. D'Amico DJ. Clinical practice. Primary retinal detachment. N Engl J Med 2008; 359:2346–54.
46. Ehrlich R, Niederer RL, Ahmad N, et al. Timing of acute macula-on rhegmatogenous retinal detachment repair. Retina 2013;33:105–10.
47. Spraul CW, Grossniklaus HE. Vitreous Hemorrhage. Surv Ophthalmol 1997;42: 3–39.
48. Micieli JA, Zurakowski D, Ahmed II. Impact of visors on eye and orbital injuries in the National Hockey League. Can J Ophthalmol 2014;49:243–8.
49. Easterbrook M. Ocular injuries in racquet sports. Int Ophthalmol Clin 1988;28: 232–7.
50. Easterbrook M. Eye injuries in squash: a preventable disease. Can Med Assoc J 1978;118:298, 303–5.
51. Easterbrook M. Prevention of eye injuries in racquet sports. Ophthalmol Clin North Am 1999;12:367–80.
52. Easterbrook M. Eye protection in racquet sports. Clin Sports Med 1988;7:253–66.
53. Napier SM, Baker RS, Sanford DG, et al. Eye injuries in athletics and recreation. Surv Ophthalmol 1996;41:229–44.

54. Micieli R, Micieli JA. Factors influencing visor use among players in the National Hockey League (NHL). Open Access J Sports Med 2014;5:43–6.
55. Easterbrook M, Devenyi R. Eye protection in professional hockey. Can J Ophthalmol 2014;49:235.
56. Micieli R, Micieli JA. Visor use among National Hockey League players and its relationship to on-ice performance. Inj Prev 2016;22(6):392–5.
57. Pashby TH. Eye injuries in hockey. Int Ophthalmol Clin 1981;21:59–86.
58. Federation of International Lacrosse. International Women's lacrosse rules. 2010. Available at: https://filacrosse.com/wp-content/themes/sportedge/downloads/FIL_womens_field_rule_book.pdf. Accessed December 17, 2016.
59. Lincoln AE, Caswell SV, Almquist JL, et al. Effectiveness of the women's lacrosse protective eyewear mandate in the reduction of eye injuries. Am J Sports Med 2012;40:611–4.
60. Easterbrook M, Pashby TJ. Eye injuries associated with war games. CMAJ 1985; 133:415–7, 419.
61. Easterbrook M, Pashby TJ. Ocular injuries and war games. Int Ophthalmol Clin 1988;28:222–4.
62. Thach AB, Ward TP, Hollifield RD, et al. Ocular injuries from paintball pellets. Ophthalmology 1999;106:533–7.
63. Felleman DJ, Van Essen DC. Distributed hierarchical processing in the primate cerebral cortex. Cereb Cortex 1991;1:1–47.
64. Ventura RE, Balcer LJ, Galetta SL, et al. Ocular motor assessment in concussion: current status and future directions. J Neurol Sci 2016;361:79–86.
65. Ventura RE, Balcer LJ, Galetta SL. The neuro-ophthalmology of head trauma. Lancet Neurol 2014;13:1006–16.
66. Ventura RE, Jancuska JM, Balcer LJ, et al. Diagnostic tests for concussion: is vision part of the puzzle? J Neuroophthalmol 2015;35:73–81.
67. Galetta K, Liu M, Leong DF, et al. The King-Devick test of rapid number naming for concussion detection: meta-analysis and systematic review of the literature. Concussion 2016. Available at: http://www.futuremedicine.com/doi/pdf/10.2217/cnc.15.8. Accessed December 17, 2016.

Sport Injuries of the Ear and Temporal Bone

L. Mariel Osetinsky, MD, Grant S. Hamilton III, MD, Matthew L. Carlson, MD*

KEYWORDS

- Sports • Trauma • Injury • Auricular • Temporal bone

KEY POINTS

- Systematic evaluation of the ear and all its anatomic subunits must be performed when investigating ear and temporal bone trauma.
- Lacerations of the pinna require meticulous multilayer repair to reduce the risk of infection and deformity.
- Auricular hematoma requires prompt drainage and application of a bolster dressing to avoid chondronecrosis and permanent deformity.
- Facial nerve function and hearing status should be investigated thoroughly and documented as soon as possible after temporal bone trauma.
- Early subspecialty referral should be obtained in patients with facial paresis, suspected sensorineural hearing loss, temporal bone fracture, suspected cerebrospinal fluid leak or suspected intracranial injury.

OVERVIEW

When the ear or temporal bone is injured, it is important to perform a thorough and systematic evaluation. If a cursory or haphazard examination is performed, it is likely that subtle signs of important injuries may be overlooked. Whenever possible, relevant details regarding the mechanism of trauma should be obtained, including high or low impact, penetrating or blunt injury, and use of protective equipment.

Owing to the complex nature of the ear and temporal bone anatomy, ear injuries can occur in many forms and the potential risks vary greatly according to the individual

Financial Material & Support: Internal departmental funding was utilized without commercial sponsorship or support.
Conflict(s) of Interest to Declare: M.L. Carlson is a consultant for MED-EL GmbH. G.S. Hamilton is a consultant for Spirox, Inc.
Institutional Review Board Approval: Not required.
Department of Otorhinolaryngology, Mayo Clinic, 200 1st Street Southwest, Rochester, MN 55905, USA
* Corresponding author. Department of Otorhinolaryngology-Head & Neck Surgery, Mayo Clinic, 200 1st Street Southwest, Rochester, MN 55905.
E-mail address: carlson.matthew@mayo.edu

sport. For example, wrestling is associated commonly with perichondritis and auricular hematoma, whereas surfing, water skiing, and kayaking are associated commonly with acute otitis externa and external auditory canal exostosis. The objective of this review is to provide the reader with a basic understanding of the relevant anatomy, evaluation, and management of sport-related injuries involving the ear and temporal bone.

RELEVANT ANATOMY OF THE EAR AND TEMPORAL BONE

Before discussing specific injury types, it is valuable to review the relevant anatomy and physiology of the ear and temporal bone. Understanding these details will provide the background necessary to appreciate the specific concerns that arise from various injuries as well as treatment considerations.

Anatomy of the External Ear

The external ear is composed of the pinna and external auditory canal. In comparison with the rest of the superficial head and neck, the skin of the ear is thin with minimal subcutaneous tissue. Similar to the surrounding scalp, neck, and face, the external ear receives a robust and redundant blood supply from several terminal branches of the external carotid artery system, including the superficial temporal artery, occipital artery, and anastomosing arteries of the scalp. The rich vascular supply of the external ear helps to explain why even simple lacerations may bleed profusely, how the ear may survive even near-complete avulsion injuries with proper management, why infection is uncommon even with gross contamination, and why primary closure can be considered in almost all cases, even several days after injury. Despite common teaching, local anesthetic injection such as 1% lidocaine with epinephrine 1:100,000 can be used safely in simple laceration repair without consequence; however, epinephrine should be avoided strictly near a tenuous vascular pedicle, as in complex lacerations or avulsions. Although the external ear has an excellent blood supply, during prolonged exposure to cold temperatures blood is shunted toward the body's core, making the ear especially prone to frostbite.[1–3]

The supporting framework of the pinna is composed of a fibroelastic cartilage, which is only absent in the fatty lobule. It is crucial to understand that the cartilage of the ear receives its blood supply solely from the overlying perichondrium and skin (**Fig. 1**).[1] Traumatic auricular hematomas develop in the subperichondrial space and deprive the underlying cartilage of critical nutrients. If not treated in a timely manner, auricular hematomas may result in long-term auricular deformity, as discussed elsewhere in this article. The cartilage of the ear is relatively thin and soft; therefore, a fine, monofilament, absorbable suture should be used to approximate cartilage edges with minimal direct handling with forceps. Repeated pinching with forceps will result in torn edges owing to the friable nature of auricular cartilage.

The lateral one-half of the ear canal is supported by cartilage and the medial one-half is encased by the temporal bone. Similar to the pinna, the skin of the ear canal is extremely thin. This is relevant for several reasons. First, external auditory canal lacerations are found commonly in the setting of longitudinal temporal bone fractures that involve the bony ear canal. This is because the thin skin of the ear canal is torn in the absence of any fatty layer to cushion it from the underlying fractured bony edges. Second, without the thermal insulation a fatty layer would provide, external auditory canal skin subjected to repetitive cold water exposure can lead to endosteal irritation and resultant focal bone growth, leading to exostosis (**Fig. 2**).

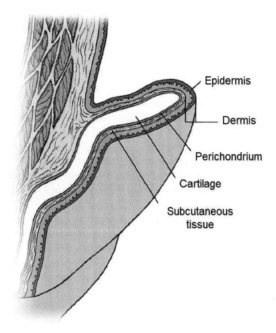

Epidermis

Dermis

Perichondrium

Cartilage

Subcutaneous
tissue

Fig. 1. Axial cross-sectional view of the layers of the external ear. When repairing an injury to the pinna, special attention must be paid to approximating the cartilage and perichondrium before approximating the overlying skin and soft tissue.

Anatomy of the Middle Ear

The tympanic membrane is anchored in the medial aperture of the ear canal and is composed of a thin, 3-layer structure. As a result, temporal bone fractures involving the ear canal commonly result in tympanic membrane laceration or perforation. The medial tympanic membrane is connected to the umbo of the malleus. The ossicular chain, composed of the malleus, incus, and stapes, is responsible for propagating the mechanical vibrations of acoustic energy from the tympanic membrane to the inner ear. The medial-most ossicle, the stapes, acts as a piston at the cochlear oval

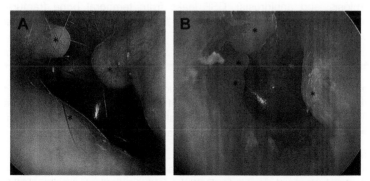

Fig. 2. (*A, B*) Exostoses (*asterisks*) in 2 patients with a history of frequent cold water exposure. Otoscopic views of the tympanic membranes are partially obstructed by multiple bony prominences emanating from the temporal bone in the medial external auditory canal.

window and creates a watertight seal between the aerated middle ear and the fluid-filled inner ear. Thus, the presence of a tympanic membrane perforation should alert the physician to the possibility of ossicular disruption, perilymphatic fistula, or inner ear injury, as described later in this article.[1,2]

Anatomy of the Inner Ear

The inner ear is composed of the cochlea, responsible for sensorineural hearing, and the labyrinth, responsible for detecting angular and linear acceleration. Injury to any portion of the ear lateral to the cochlea may result in conductive hearing loss, whereas injury to the inner ear may result in sensorineural hearing loss or vestibular symptoms. Because the otic capsule is composed of the densest bone of the body, only a small percentage of temporal bone fractures involve the inner ear.[1] However, the cochlea and vestibule contain very delicate neuromembranous structures and, therefore, fractures of the otic capsule nearly always result in profound hearing loss and vestibular hypofunction. Furthermore, the fluid of the inner ear is in continuity with the intracranial subarachnoid space, and therefore fractures of the otic capsule may result in a cerebrospinal fluid (CSF) leak and meningitis. The otic capsule is also notably unique in the sense that fractures heal with incomplete union, and neo-ossification does not occur. As a result, delayed meningitis can occur in the absence of an obvious CSF leak, even years after injury.[1,4,5]

Facial Nerve

Of all the cranial nerves, the facial nerve has the longest course through the skull base—traversing the narrow fallopian canal. The facial nerve enters the temporal bone at the fundus of the internal auditory canal and follows a convoluted course through the temporal bone to reach the stylomastoid foramen, where it exits the skull near the temporomandibular joint, and branches into 5 divisions at the pes anserinus within the parotid gland before its many branches innervate the muscles of facial expression (**Fig. 3**).

Lateral Skull Base

The lateral skull base is composed of the temporal, occipital, and sphenoid bones and contains numerous coursing neurovascular structures. Injury to the lateral skull base may result in a CSF leak, intracranial bleed, cranial neuropathy, and other sequelae. Because sympathetic innervation of the head and eye courses along the adventitia of the internal carotid artery, patients with internal carotid artery injury within the temporal bone (eg, pseudoaneurysm, dissection) may present with Horner's syndrome (ptosis, miosis, and anhidrosis). CSF leaks from temporal bone fractures most commonly result from fracturing of the thin "roof" or tegmen of the middle ear or mastoid.[1,5]

PHYSICAL EXAMINATION

Only after the primary trauma evaluation should a focused examination of the ear and temporal bone be performed. The ear and all of its anatomic subunits should be examined, including the periauricular region and scalp, auricle, external auditory canal, tympanic membrane, middle ear, inner ear, cranial nerves and carotid artery.

- Periauricular region and scalp
  - Soft tissue laceration, contusion, or hematoma.
  - Postauricular ecchymosis (ie, Battle's sign) may indicate basilar skull fracture.
  - Preauricular, facial, or neck laceration risks facial nerve transection or contusion.

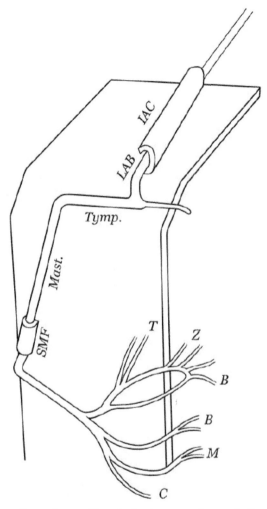

Fig. 3. Facial nerve pathway from exiting the brainstem at the cerebellopontine angle (*top*) to distal branches (*bottom*). The nerve can be injured anywhere along this course. Related to head or ear trauma, indirect injury to the nerve leading to swelling within its restrictive bony canal within the temporal bone (IAC to stylomastoid foramen) can cause vascular ischemia and congestion resulting in facial weakness. Weakness can also be caused by direct injury to facial nerve fibers by fractured bone or penetrating trauma. BB, buccal branches; C, cervical branch; IAC, internal auditory canal; LAB, labyrinthine segment; M, marginal mandibular branch; Mast, mastoid segment; SMF, stylomastoid foramen; T, temporal branch; Tymp, tympanic segment; Z, zygomatic branch.

- Auricle
  - Laceration, avulsion, or hematoma.
  - Edema with loss of contour may indicate perichondritis or early hematoma formation.
  - Fluctuance indicates hematoma, seroma, or abscess development.
- External auditory canal
  - Edema, narrowing of the external auditory canal, and pain may indicate otitis externa.

- ○ Sessile bony protrusions (ie, exostoses) may indicate repetitive exposure to cold water.
  - ○ Bloody otorrhea or laceration may indicate underlying temporal bone fracture.
  - ○ Clear or serosanguineous otorrhea may indicate CSF leak.
- Tympanic membrane
  - ○ Tympanic membrane perforation raises concern for middle or inner ear injury or temporal bone fracture.
- Middle ear
  - ○ Hemotympanum raises concern for temporal bone fracture.
  - ○ Malrotation of the malleus may indicate ossicular disruption.
- Inner ear
  - ○ Direct examination of the inner ear is not possible with otoscopy; however, spontaneous horizontal nystagmus or asymmetrical sensorineural hearing loss, determined using a Weber tuning fork test, may indicate inner ear injury.
- Cranial nerves and carotid artery
  - ○ Abducens nerve (cranial nerve VI).
    - ■ Ipsilateral lateral gaze palsy may indicate intracranial injury, or basilar skull fracture involving the anterior petrous temporal bone or region of the cavernous sinus.[5,6]
  - ○ Facial nerve (cranial nerve VII)
    - ■ Paresis or paralysis of the ipsilateral hemiface may indicate intracranial injury (rare), temporal bone fracture (more common), or extratemporal soft tissue injury.[2]
    - ■ Documenting the timing of paralysis (ie, immediate or delayed) and severity (ie, partial or complete paralysis) is critical in predicting the outcome and potential need for treatment.
  - ○ Lower cranial nerves (cranial nerve IX-XII)
    - ■ Paresis or paralysis from sport injuries is rare but may indicate intracranial, temporal bone, jugular foramen, or extratemporal trauma.[5,6]
  - ○ Carotid artery
    - ■ Internal carotid artery injury from temporal bone trauma is rare and may present with ipsilateral Horner's syndrome (ie, lid ptosis, miosis, and anhidrosis), symptoms of stroke, or, rarely, massive bloody otorrhea.[5,6]

SPECIFIC TYPES OF INJURY: EVALUATION AND MANAGEMENT
Auricular Soft Tissue Trauma

Soft tissue injuries are among the most common forms of trauma sustained by the ear during sport activities and can be caused by a number of mechanisms. Furthermore, auricular injuries can present in a variety of ways with variable tissue involvement, requiring a corresponding degree of complexity in medical and surgical management. The primary types of soft tissue injury involving the external ear that are discussed in this section include abrasions, lacerations, and avulsions. Auricular hematomas are discussed in detail in a section to follow.

The basic tenets of wound management are particularly important in managing auricular soft tissue trauma. A review of the patient's immunization record and need for tetanus prophylaxis or booster should be assessed in all cases. The choice of preparatory solution for surgical field cleaning is important. Betadine (10% povidone-iodine) is inexpensive, readily available at most centers, and is not ototoxic. If the patient does not have an iodine allergy, betadine is an excellent choice for cleaning the ear. The use of 4% chlorhexidine gluconate (Hibiclens, Mölnlycke Health

Care, Norcross, GA) must be strictly avoided because this solution is ototoxic and may enter the middle ear space if a perforation is present. Copious irrigation is critical in preventing posttraumatic auricular chondritis or other infectious complications. Careful attention should be paid while irrigating the wound to identify and remove any visible debris. Sterile saline is another good option for irrigation because this solution will not risk soft tissue irritation and is not ototoxic. Irrigation with an antibiotic solution is acceptable; however, the treating physician must use caution to avoid irrigating any traumatic ear wound with an ototoxic medication such as gentamicin or neomycin.

Perioperative intravenous or oral antibiotic prophylaxis is beneficial, particularly with cartilage exposure or gross contamination. Antibiotics effective against *Pseudomonas* spp. such as levofloxacin or ciprofloxacin are recommended for prophylaxis against auricular chondritis. The one caveat to this is the risk of tendonitis and Achilles tendon rupture in the pediatric population. This risk may be greater in athletes and other active patients.

Auricular abrasion

Auricular abrasions are defined by a shearing injury of the epidermal and superficial dermal layers without loss or separation of the deeper dermal or subdermal components. If any amount of cartilage is involved, the injury may be described more accurately as an "auricular avulsion" injury. Auricular abrasions can occur in sports such as boxing or wrestling, with a quick blow by a gloved hand or against a training mat. Artificial turf is another common cause of auricular abrasions in field sports, as can pavement as in the case of biking, skateboarding, or luge accidents.

Proper management of auricular abrasion is similar to management of abrasion injuries involving other parts of the body. Petroleum jelly can act as a protective barrier in the healing of an abrasion. One should use caution with certain antibiotic ointments, because antimicrobials such as neomycin can be ototoxic. Furthermore, up to 22% of patients may experience local irritation or contact dermatitis from common topical antibiotic ointments, resulting in erythema, which may be mistaken for secondary infection.[7] Vaseline promotes healing by protecting the injured tissue from the external environment, as well as moisturizing the newly granulating tissue by acting as an occlusive dressing.

Auricular laceration

An auricular laceration describes a transection of the soft tissue of the ear without a loss of any full-thickness tissue segment (**Fig. 4**). Auricular lacerations are repaired through primary closure with sutures. Laceration can involve any of the anatomic components of the auricle, from the cartilage-bearing subunits of the pinna to the skin and subcutaneous fatty tissue of the lobule. Contact with a sharp or high-velocity object such as a fish hook, knife, tree branch, ski edge, skate blade, fingernail, or tooth can cause auricular laceration injuries. Earrings are commonly caught and pulled in sporting events, causing a tear in the lobule.

The same basic principles of soft tissue injury management apply when caring for patients with auricular laceration: irrigation, removal of foreign bodies, tissue approximation, and antibiotic prophylaxis. After the wound has been cleaned thoroughly, repair of the laceration can begin. It is critical that the ear be closed approximating all anatomic layers. Typically, 5-0 sutures are appropriate for closure. Approximation of the perichondrial layer and cartilage edges with simple interrupted absorbable monofilament suture should be performed first (see **Fig. 1**). Ear cartilage is soft and easily fractures with frequent handling; therefore, minimal manipulation of the cartilage

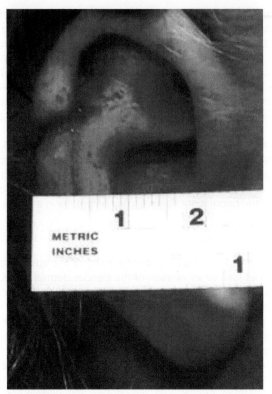

Fig. 4. Full-thickness auricular laceration. For proper healing and avoidance of chondritis or chondronecrosis, the cartilage and perichondrium must be handled carefully and all layers must be reapproximated meticulously.

should be performed and the cartilage should never be handled with a toothed forceps. After this, closure of the skin and subcutaneous tissue can begin with simple interrupted 5-0 or 6-0 suture. Beyond better wound approximation, an advantage of simple interrupted sutures over running sutures is the opportunity for any residual blood or other fluid to drain out of the wound through the gaps between interrupted sutures, decreasing the risk for posttraumatic auricular hematoma or seroma. The goal of soft tissue closure is approximation without strangulation—the final layer of sutures should evert the skin gently and should not be overly tight.

When using an absorbable suture in the skin, there may be a period of prolonged inflammation around the margins of the wound. However, a considerable benefit of repairing an auricular soft tissue injury with absorbable suture material is to obviate the need for the patient to return to the clinic for suture removal. Retained sutures or improper suture removal performed outside the health care setting may lead to infection or poor wound healing for the patient. If the patient is able to return for suture removal, using a monofilament material will lead to a better looking wound faster, owing to the decreased inflammation.

Auricular avulsion

Avulsion is a severe transection injury resulting in complete or near-complete separation of soft tissue from its native site. The aforementioned principles of wound management apply to auricular avulsion. However, the added complexity of maintaining soft tissue vitality becomes critical. All avulsed segments of an auricle should be retrieved and transported with the patient whenever possible. During transport, the detached segments can be stored in room temperature to slightly cool normal saline; however, clean water can suffice if normal saline is not available. There are limited data in the literature to claim the single best transport medium for an avulsed auricle in preparation for reattachment, but there have been reports of successful replantation of large auricular segments transported on ice baths, even in some cases of auricular fragments retrieved from the scene hours after the injury.[8–11]

There are 4 approaches that can be undertaken when confronted with auricular avulsion: leave the defect unrepaired, primary closure without incorporating the segment of avulsed tissue, reattachment of the avulsed segment, and postauricular pocketing of denuded auricular cartilage with delayed harvest.[9–11]

1. *Leave the defect unrepaired.* This is the simplest approach and can be used when the avulsed tissue is unrecoverable or unsuitable for use. This strategy generally results in a noticeable deformity and is not advisable in most cases.
2. *Primary closure without incorporating the segment of avulsed tissue.* This technique may be accomplished through local advancement or rotational flaps, or, very rarely, grafts from the contralateral ear. Examples include wedge or stellate excision with closure or advancement of the helical rim. Similar to the first option, this strategy may be used when the avulsed tissue is not available for unsuitable for reattachment. However, in many cases, this approach can result in an acceptable appearance, provided the defect is not large.
3. *Reattachment of the avulsed segment* (**Fig. 5**). In the author's opinion, this strategy should be used in essentially every case of incomplete avulsion (ie, a vascular pedicle is preserved) and in most cases where suitable tissue is available. With incomplete avulsion, microvascular perfusion can be assessed by warmth of the tissue, the presence and briskness of capillary refill, and the existence of punctate bleeding at the leading edge of the partially avulsed segment. Even complete avulsion injuries have a chance of integration, and in the worst case the devitalized segment will necrose and the physician can default to the second option. To repair an auricular avulsion injury when all segments have been recovered, the same principles of auricular laceration repair should be applied with special added attention to preservation of microvasculature — minimal to no cautery should be used at the leading edges of the wound, no vasoconstrictor should be injected, cold irrigation should not be used, sutures should be placed further apart and should not be overly tight, and compression from a wound dressing should be avoided. Steffen and colleagues[11] advocate for microvascular anastomosis of auricular avulsion injuries when feasible; however, finding a suitable and appropriately size-matched artery and vein on the avulsed side can be highly challenging and is usually not possible.[2] Others including Kalus[9] describe excellent outcomes without microvascular anastomosis in repairing complete auricular avulsion. Good reperfusion of reattached tissue can be achieved with a clean well-approximated 3-layered repair.

Relevant to this topic, 2 strategies can be considered when concerned with severe microvascular compromise. First, hyperbaric oxygen therapy improves oxygen diffusion, enhances tissue perfusion, promotes healing, and carries bactericidal effects.[10] Second, even with good arterial reperfusion, venous congestion may occur, presenting with edema and purple discoloration. In these cases, leech therapy may be considered. Not only does leech therapy assist with clearing venous pooling, but leech saliva

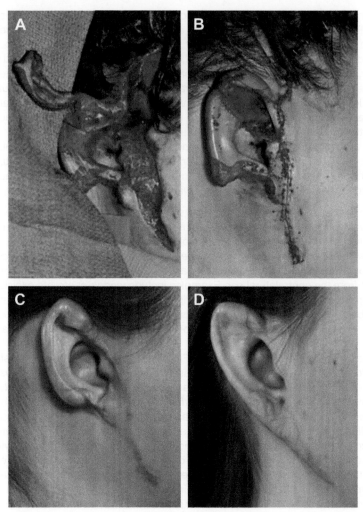

Fig. 5. Complex auricular avulsion involving helical rim and lobe, as well as complex preauricular laceration: before repair (*A*), immediately after primary repair (*B*), 3 months later (*C*), and after revision surgery with full-thickness skin graft to fill the soft tissue deficit at the earlobe (*D*).

contains the protein hirudin, a potent anticoagulant that may act to mitigate arterial and venous thrombosis.[1,2,11]

4. *Postauricular pocketing of denuded auricular cartilage with delayed harvest* (**Fig. 6**). If a large segment of the cartilage-bearing auricle has been avulsed completely, or in the case of total external ear avulsion, the cartilage framework may be salvaged by removing the overlying skin and placing the cartilage framework in a subcutaneous postauricular pocket. Recall that auricular cartilage depends the blood supply of the surrounding perichondrium and skin, thus, this strategy may salvage the avulsed segment of cartilage, which is critical to the shape of the ear and technically difficult to replicate with rib cartilage carving or nonautologous implants.

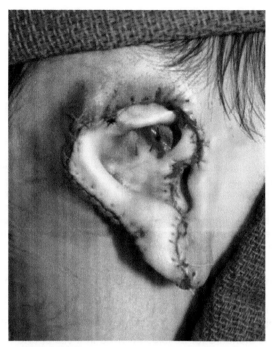

Fig. 6. Auricular avulsion after first stage of multistep repair. In this figure, auricular carti-lage is "banked" in a postauricular soft tissue pocket that provides donor skin with improved vascular supply. Auricular cartilage is banked for several weeks to months before elevating the auricle in a multistage repair.

Auricular Hematoma

Blunt or shearing trauma to the ear, such as can be sustained by a boxing glove or in a wrestling match, can lead to the formation of an auricular hematoma (**Figs. 7** and **8**). Auricular hematoma refers to a collection of blood in the subperichondrial space of the external ear, depriving the underlying cartilage of nutrients. Appropriate early manage-ment of this common sport injury is important in preventing abscess formation and permanent deformities of the pinna.

The anatomy of the auricle is such that auricular hematomas occur almost exclu-sively on the anterior surface of the pinna. The subcutaneous fatty layer on the poste-rior auricle is somewhat protective against traumatic shearing forces. On the anterior surface of the auricle, however, there is little to no subcutaneous fatty layer; instead, the skin is immediately adherent to the perichondrium. Therefore, when a strong shearing force is applied to the auricle, the posterior auricular skin easily slides over the perichondrium. However, with this same force applied to the anterior surface of the ear, a tear in the perichondrium may occur, resulting in subperichondrial hema-toma development. When blood collects in the potential space between the cartilage and the perichondrium, a clot results, creating a barrier to nutrient transfer. If not drained, acute chondronecrosis ensues, leading eventually to a permanent dense fibrotic deformity of the pinna known as "cauliflower ear" (see **Figs. 7** and **8**).

An auricular hematoma can be identified by loss of the folds of the pinna and underlying fluctuance. Once the diagnosis has been established, the focus of the sur-geon should be to drain the fluid collection as soon as possible. The ideal timing of

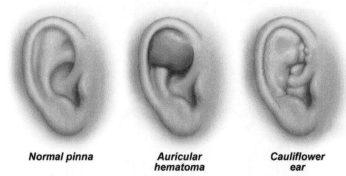

Normal pinna   **Auricular hematoma**   **Cauliflower ear**

Fig. 7. Development of auricular hematoma and subsequent cauliflower ear deformity. In the acute setting, an auricular hematoma is a fluctuant red or purple swelling on the anterior pinna. Without proper intervention, a fibrotic scar forms where the fluid collection once was. This gives rise to a deformity known as "cauliflower ear," which is commonly seen among boxers and wrestlers.

drainage is within the first 5 to 7 days; however, early drainage within the first 1 or 2 days is ideal.

As with all medical conditions, prevention is the priority. Particular sports, including boxing and wrestling, are known to have an high incidence of auricular hematoma. It has nearly become standard for athletes involved in these sports to wear protective equipment to avoid such injuries.

Procedure for drainage of auricular hematoma

There are multiple methods of draining an auricular hematoma. Regardless of the approach, several underlying principles should be observed including early drainage, adequate bolstering in the postdrainage period to prevent reaccumulation, and antimicrobial prophylaxis. Follow-up within 1 week should always take place to remove the bolster dressing and to confirm adequate drainage.

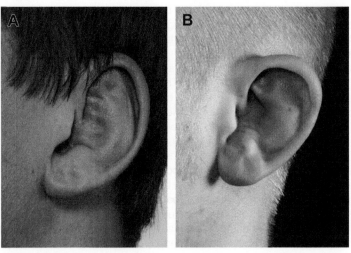

Fig. 8. Auricular hematoma (*A*) and cauliflower ear deformity (*B*), which forms after inadequate drainage of an auricular hematoma.

The most common method used by the authors is as follows.

1. First, the auricle is anesthetized. This maneuver can be performed using either direct local injection of 1% lidocaine or a local nerve block. If an auricular block is performed, special caution should be used when injecting below the tragus anteriorly or below the mastoid tip posteriorly because temporary facial nerve paresis can occur.
2. After adequate local anesthesia is achieved, the ear is prepped sterilely with betadine.
3. Using an 11-blade, a curvilinear incision is made superficially where the concave surfaces of the anterior pinna would normally be (**Fig. 9**). This often requires 2 separate incisions, 1 incision between the helix and antihelix in the scaphoid fossa and 1 incision in the conchal bowl.
4. All clot and fluid should be evacuated thoroughly with pressure followed by copious irrigation.
5. A bolster dressing is then prepared. The authors prefer using dental rolls on either side of the helix and antihelix (anteriorly and posteriorly), secured with a 2-0 or 0-0 nylon suture thrown in a horizontal mattress fashion, and Xeroform in the conchal

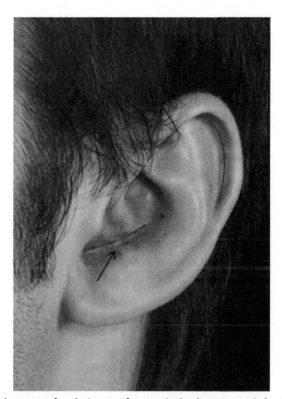

Fig. 9. Incision placement for drainage of an auricular hematoma is best situated in the dependent portion of the fluid collection and following the curvature of the concave surface of the pinna (*dotted lines*). In this figure, a discrete scar (*arrow*) is visible from a previously placed incision made for drainage of a hematoma that was involving the conchal bowl. After proper drainage and bolster placement, the normal anatomic features of the pinna remain intact.

bowl. The bolster should be snug, to prevent reaccumulation, but not overly tight, to avoid necrosis. The authors advocate for oral antibiotic coverage while the bolster dressing is in place for 5 days. On day 5, the patient should return to the clinic for removal of the bolster dressing and for careful evaluation of the pinna to inspect for necrosis, recollection, or infection.

Otitis Externa

Otitis externa, commonly referred to as "swimmer's ear," is an infection of the soft tissue of the external auditory canal. Common causative pathogens include *Pseudomonas aeruginosa*, *Staphylococcus epidermidis*, and *Staphylococcus aureus*; less commonly, fungal infections may occur.[3] Patient factors that predispose athletes to otitis externa include exposure to damp environments, exposure to natural sources of nonchlorinated water, narrow ear canals, and exostoses or other obstructions. Presenting symptoms of ear pain, purulent drainage, swollen or erythematous ear canals, or pruritus should raise the clinician's suspicion for otitis externa. Tragal tenderness on palpation and pain with gentle posterior traction of the pinna are hallmark physical examination findings. Treatment includes ear wick placement, particularly for already stenotic or edematous ear canals, and initiation of a 7-day course of an ototopical antimicrobial agent with or without a steroid component. Additional oral antibiotics are reserved typically for cases in which there is concern for the ability of ototopical drops to access the medial ear canal or if there is any evidence of a developing malignant otitis externa.

Frostbite

The ears are prone to both cold injuries and thermal burns owing to their vulnerable location. Cold injuries most commonly present with pain, swelling, and redness, and should be treated cautiously with rewarming in the acute setting. According to Hill and colleagues,[2] rapid rewarming over 30 minutes with a 40°C solution is the single most important predictor of tissue salvage in patients with frostbite.[3] This process is exquisitely painful to the patient and should be managed appropriately with narcotic analgesics as needed. Only after the rewarming process is entirely complete can the state of the injured tissue be assessed accurately. Hill and colleagues also suggest the extent of a frostbite injury of the ears before warming may seem to be either deceptively better or worse than the true state of the frostbitten tissue after proper thermal recovery. After initial supportive therapy and careful assessment, next-line treatments can include antibiotic prophylaxis such as with a penicillin, scheduled ibuprofen, and hyperbaric oxygen to salvage any viable tissue. The authors discourage surgical debridement in the acute setting, because tissue affected by frostbite wounds can take weeks to declare ultimate viability.[3]

Exostosis

Exostosis refers to the development of sessile bony protuberances in the medial ear canal that result from repetitive cold water exposure, such as with ocean surfing, kayaking, or cold water swimming.[3] In most cases, exostoses occur bilaterally, with multiple separate lesions in either ear (see **Fig. 2**). It is theorized that repetitive cold water exposure results in irritation of the underlying bone that is particularly vulnerable owing to the paper-thin skin of the medial ear canal without fatty thermal insulation. In most cases, no treatment is required. However, large growths may result in recurrent otitis externa, medial trapping of ear canal debris, or conductive hearing loss and may require surgical intervention by an otologist.

Temporal Bone Fractures

Temporal bone fractures may occur after a direct forceful blow to the temporal or occipital skull. Temporal bone fractures have traditionally been described as either "longitudinal" or "transverse," according to the direction of the fracture line in relation to the axis of the petrous temporal bone (**Figs. 10** and **11**). Longitudinal fractures, which run parallel to the petrous ridge, are the most common type of temporal bone fracture (80%) and are usually caused by a temporal blow. In contrast, transverse fractures, perpendicular to the petrous ridge, are less common (20%) and usually result from blunt occipital trauma. Although this traditional method of classifying fractures as either longitudinal or transverse is still widely used, an updated and more clinically relevant way to categorize temporal bone fractures has gained popularity by referring to the level of otic capsule involvement. Longitudinal fractures are less likely to involve the otic capsule and typically spare the facial nerve. Alternatively, transverse fractures are more likely to involve the otic capsule, resulting in sensorineural hearing loss, and more commonly result in facial paresis. Nevertheless, both longitudinal and transverse temporal bone fractures are capable of involving the otic capsule. A temporal bone fracture with both longitudinal and transverse components can instead be designated as "mixed" or "oblique."[1,6] A comparison of features between types of temporal bone fractures according to the different classification systems is outlined in **Tables 1** and **2**.

A laceration within the ear canal or tympanic membrane, hemotympanum, facial nerve paralysis, nystagmus, sensorineural hearing loss, or postauricular ecchymosis may indicate the presence of a basilar skull fracture. In all cases where a temporal bone or basilar skull fracture is suspected, imaging is critical to establish a diagnosis and characterize the fracture pattern. Imaging is also critical to evaluate for associated intracranial injury, pneumocephalus that may indicate CSF leak (**Fig. 12**), or involvement of the carotid canal. All patients with temporal bone fracture should be evaluated early after injury for hearing loss using a bedside Weber and Rinne 512-Hz tuning fork test. Ideally, one should perform an audiogram because it is generally perceived that the outcome of traumatic sensorineural hearing loss is better if steroids are initiated early. Conductive hearing loss from external auditory canal laceration, tympanic membrane

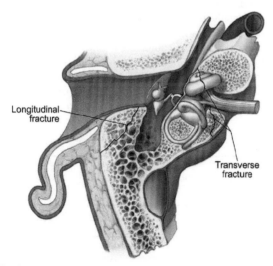

Fig. 10. Longitudinal and transverse temporal bone fractures. In this example, the longitudinal fracture is otic capsule sparing while the transverse fracture is otic capsule involving.

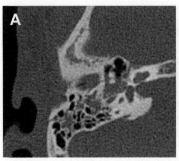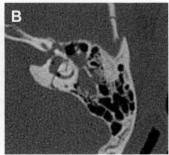

Fig. 11. Temporal bone fractures on axial computed tomography imaging. (A) Right-sided longitudinal temporal bone fracture extending from mastoid cortex, through mastoid air cells, involving the posterior external auditory canal, and extending into the middle ear. (B) Left-sided transverse temporal bone fracture in the same patient (opposite ear), involving the otic capsule at the level of the semicircular canals.

perforation, middle ear fluid, or ossicular disruption will result in a Weber test that lateralizes to the affected ear. In contrast, with sensorineural hearing loss, the Weber test lateralizes to the contralateral ear, and in that same ear, air conduction should be greater than bone conduction with the Rinne test. In most cases, an uncomplicated temporal bone fracture can be managed with strict water precautions, a short course of ototopical antibiotic drops, and follow-up with an audiogram in 6 to 12 weeks.[5,6]

The diagnosis of CSF leak in the setting of temporal bone trauma deserves special discussion, because an unrecognized leak risks the development of meningitis.[4,5,12] In the acute period, a CSF leak may be difficult to diagnose because CSF is generally mixed with blood, thereby acquiring a bloody or serosanguineous appearance. However, with time CSF otorrhea or rhinorrhea will generally become clearer, ultimately acquiring the appearance and viscosity of water. In the case of CSF rhinorrhea from temporal bone fracture, fluid should drain preferentially from the ipsilateral nostril when leaning forward (ie, Dandy maneuver). Whenever a CSF leak is suspected, external auditory canal or nasal drainage should be collected and tested for beta-2 transferrin. With a sensitivity and specificity approaching 100%, this test is highly reliable when even a small quantity of fluid can be obtained. Many texts will refer to the presence of a halo sign (ie, outer clear ring around central area of blood) as an indicator of traumatic CSF leak; however, this test is unreliable.[2,5,6] Fortunately, the great majority of traumatic CSF leaks resolve with conservative measures; however, once diagnosed, an otolaryngologist or neurosurgeon should be consulted immediately to determine and direct appropriate conservative or surgical interventions.

Table 1	
Temporal bone fracture characteristics by type	
Longitudinal	**Transverse**
80% of all temporal bone fractures	20% of all temporal bone fractures
Parallel to petrous ridge	Perpendicular to petrous ridge
Facial weakness rare	Facial weakness more common
Otic capsule involvement rare	Otic capsule involvement more common
Sensorineural hearing loss rare	Sensorineural hearing loss more common

Table 2
Temporal bone fracture characteristics by otic capsule involvement

Otic Capsule Sparing	Otic Capsule Involving
More commonly longitudinal	More commonly transverse
Conductive/mixed hearing loss	Sensorineural hearing loss
Lower risk of CSF leak	Up to 8× greater risk of CSF leak
Lower risk of intracranial complications	Greater risk of intracranial complications and delayed meningitis
Lower risk of facial nerve weakness	Greater risk of facial nerve weakness
More commonly involve external auditory canal	Rarely disrupt ossicles or external auditory canal
Temporoparietal trauma	Occipital trauma

Abbreviation: CSF, cerebrospinal fluid.

Facial Nerve Injury

Early diagnosis of traumatic facial nerve paralysis is important because prompt management may improve outcome.[5] In an alert and cooperative patient, facial weakness can be obvious to the observer through asking the patient to smile, blink, or raise their eyebrows. However, in the case of a patient who is disoriented or has a mild weakness, a unilateral facial palsy may go undetected initially. Therefore, in any case of ear or head trauma, a focused facial nerve examination should always be performed and the findings carefully documented.

Injury to the nerve can occur at any location along this path from brainstem to cutaneous muscles (see **Fig. 3**). An acute displaced temporal bone fracture through the fallopian canal typically results in immediate, complete facial nerve paralysis with

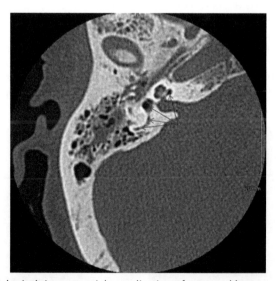

Fig. 12. Pneumolabyrinth is a potential complication of temporal bone trauma. Red arrows denote air pathologically filling the normally fluid-filled cochlea and vestibular labyrinth of the inner ear. (*Courtesy of* Alex D Sweeney, MD, Department of Otolaryngology-Head and Neck Surgery, Baylor College of Medicine, Houston, TX.)

less chance of satisfactory recovery. Delayed weakness or incomplete paresis generally occurs from a nondisplaced fracture causing neuronal edema with resultant vascular compromise within the tight confines of the bony canal. The most common location of facial nerve injury in the setting of temporal bone fractures is the perigeniculate region.[5,6] Incomplete or delayed onset facial nerve weakness generally portends a good long-term prognosis. In the majority of cases, the patient regains normal facial nerve function over the course of months. The management of acute complete facial nerve injury from temporal bone trauma is complex and may require specialized electromyographic testing, which is beyond the scope of this article. In such cases, a dedicated temporal bone computed tomography scan should be obtained, strict eye care must be maintained to avoid catastrophic corneal drying, high-dose oral glucocorticoid therapy should be initiated (unless contraindicated), and a referral to an otologist should be obtained as soon as possible because the outcome of a potential surgical intervention depends on early action.

Tympanic Membrane Perforation

Traumatic tympanic membrane perforation (**Fig. 13**) may occur in a variety of ways, including temporal bone fracture, penetrating trauma (eg, tree branch), barotrauma (eg, scuba diving, altitude change, and hand or water slap to ear), or blast injuries. The majority of traumatic perforations heal without intervention (**Fig. 14**); however, deeper injuries should be considered and evaluated properly. If it is determined that an isolated tympanic membrane injury occurred, then the patient should be instructed to maintain dry ear precautions (ie, no water in the ear canal), a course of ototopical antibiotic drops should be prescribed, and the patient should follow-up with an otolaryngologist to ensure the tympanic membrane heals and no long-term sequelae develop such as cholesteatoma.

Perilymphatic Fistula

The inner ear contains an ionically balanced fluid called perilymph. Disruption of the stapes footplate at the oval window, or tearing of the round window membrane may result in a perilymphatic fistula with fluid leakage into the middle ear. The mechanism of traumatic perilymphatic fistula involves direct disruption from temporal bone fracture, or high energy transmitted pressure from barotrauma. Symptoms of perilymphatic fistula include fluctuating or sudden sensorineural hearing loss, and Valsalva-induced vertigo.[5,6] In severe cases, temporal bone computed tomography scanning

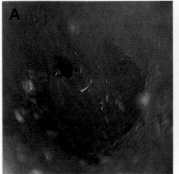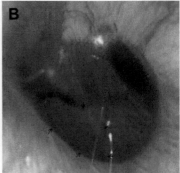

Fig. 13. Traumatic tympanic membrane perforations (*A, B*). Arrows delineate the edges of the perforations.

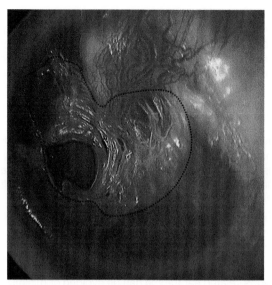

Fig. 14. Tympanic membrane actively healing (*thin dashed line*) 3 weeks after incurring a large traumatic perforation (*thick dotted line*).

may demonstrate disruption of the ossicular chain and stapes footplate or pneumolabyrinth (see **Fig. 12**); however, in many cases the diagnosis may be elusive and requires an high index of suspicion. Patients with perilymphatic fistula are generally treated with oral glucocorticoids, placed on bedrest or light activity, and given stool softeners to avoid potentiating perilymphatic drainage. More severe cases may be managed successfully with middle ear exploration and "patching" of the oval or round window membranes.[5,6]

Acoustic Trauma

Exposure to loud or repeated noise is an important risk factor for sensorineural hearing loss. Sports activities involving firearms or high-powered engines place certain athletes at risk for developing sensorineural hearing loss over time.[13,14] Noise-induced hearing loss can be demonstrated audiometrically by a threshold shift in pure tone hearing. Threshold shifts as an indicator of hearing loss can be either temporary or permanent. In patients with a recent history of noise exposure complaining of hearing loss, audiometry should be performed in the acute setting. If sensorineural hearing loss is identified in a patient with recent noise exposure who complains of new hearing loss, a steroid burst and taper should be prescribed in an attempt to salvage hearing. In cases of permanent hearing loss, options for rehabilitation include conventional hearing aids, contralateral routing of signal aids, bone conduction hearing aids, and cochlear implantation, depending on the severity of hearing loss and the status of hearing in the opposite ear.[14] Wearing hearing protection with ear plugs or muffs can help to mitigate the risk of noise-induced hearing loss in all patients, particularly those exposed to loud or repetitive equipment and machinery at work or in sports.[15]

Labyrinthine Concussion

Just as head trauma can lead to cerebral concussion, trauma to the ear and temporal bone can cause a concussive process involving the structures of the inner ear.

Labyrinthine concussion may result in temporary or permanent sensorineural hearing loss or vestibular dysfunction. Patients will often report acute hearing loss and vertigo and on examination they may exhibit horizontal nystagmus. A high-resolution temporal bone computed tomography scan is required to distinguish labyrinthine concussion from otic capsule fracture. Oral glucocorticoid therapy should be considered for treatment.[5,6]

SPECIAL CONSIDERATIONS

Patients born with inner ear malformations, such as enlarged vestibular aqueduct, can suffer from permanent hearing loss with even a minor head injury. Patients with enlarged vestibular aqueduct are often without syndromic features and may be born with normal hearing leading to a delay in diagnosis. If an individual is known to have an enlarged vestibular aqueduct or other inner ear malformation, they should be informed regarding the risks of hearing loss from participating in contact sports and other higher risk activities or careers.[16–19]

PREVENTION

In many cases, sports-related ear trauma can be avoided or minimized with adequate preventive measures. Protective head gear is considered standard in certain high-impact sports such as football, boxing, and wrestling. Baseball players wear helmets to protect against errant pitches or stray swings of the bat, which have been known to cause temporal bone fractures. Exostoses, bony overgrowths of the external auditory canal, can be avoided in scuba divers and surfers by wearing swimmers' ear plugs or special caps while exposed to colder waters.

Because repetitive loud noise exposure is a known risk factor for progressive sensorineural hearing loss, hearing protection should be worn by pilots, race car drivers, hunters, sharpshooters, and other athletes exposed to significant levels of noise. Although hearing loss is not linked commonly to sports injuries, the effects of repetitive or sustained noise exposure predisposes patients to progressive irreversible hearing loss later in life and thus noise exposure should be limited by protective wear whenever possible.[15]

SUMMARY

Ear trauma can manifest in many ways. Soft tissue injuries, hearing loss, and temporal bone fractures require vastly different approaches to diagnosis and treatment. Although the initial workup may be performed in an emergency department or by a primary care doctor, consultation with an otolaryngologist, plastic surgeon, or neurosurgeon will add valuable specialty experience.

REFERENCES

1. Francis HW. Anatomy of the temporal bone, external ear, and middle ear. In: Flint PW, Haughey BH, Lund V, et al, editors. Cummings Otolaryngology head and neck surgery. 6th edition. Philadelphia: Elsevier Saunders; 2015. p. 1977–86.
2. Hill JD, Stoddard DG, Hamilton GS. Facial trauma. In: Flint PW, Haughey BH, Lund V, et al, editors. Cummings Otolaryngology head and neck surgery. 6th edition. Philadelphia: Elsevier Saunders; 2015. p. 307–24.
3. Öztürkcan S, Öztürkcan S. Dermatologic diseases of the external ear. Clin Dermatol 2014;32(1):141–52.

4. Bernal-Sprekelsen M, Bleda-Vázquez C, Carrau RL. Ascending meningitis secondary to traumatic cerebrospinal fluid leaks. Am J Rhinol 2000;14(4):257–9.
5. Brodie HA, Thompson TC. Management of complications from 820 temporal bone fractures. Am J Otolaryngol 1997;18(2):188–97.
6. Brodie HA, Wilkerson BJ. Management of temporal bone trauma. In: Flint PW, Haughey BH, Lund V, et al, editors. Cummings Otolaryngology head and neck surgery. 6th edition. Philadelphia: Elsevier Saunders; 2015. p. 2220–32.
7. Jacob SE, James WD. From road rash to top allergen in a flash: bacitracin. Dermatol Surg 2004;30(4):521–4.
8. Emerich K, Kaczmarek J. First aid for dental trauma caused by sports activities. Sports Med 2010;40(5):361–6.
9. Kalus R. Successful bilateral composite ear reattachment. Plast Reconstr Surg Glob Open 2014;2(6):e174.
10. Rapley JH, Lawrence WT, Witt PD. Composite grafting and hyperbaric oxygen therapy in pediatric nasal tip reconstruction after avulsive dog-bite injury. Ann Plast Surg 2001;46(4):434–8.
11. Steffen A, Katzbach R, Klaiber S. A comparison of ear reattachment methods: a review of 25 years since Pennington. Plast Reconstr Surg 2006;118(6):1358–64.
12. Kamochi H, Kusaka G, Ishikawa M, et al. Late onset cerebrospinal fluid leakage associated with past head injury. Neurol Med Chir (Tokyo) 2013;53(4):217–20.
13. Irgens-Hansen K, Sunde E, Bråtveit M, et al. Hearing loss in the royal Norwegian navy: a cross-sectional study. Int Arch Occup Environ Health 2014;88(5):641–9.
14. Lonsbury-Martin BL, Martin GK. Noise-induced hearing loss. In: Flint PW, Haughey BH, Lund V, et al, editors. Cummings Otolaryngology head and neck surgery. 6th edition. Philadelphia: Elsevier Saunders; 2015. p. 2345–58.
15. Ramakers GG, Kraaijenga VJC, Cattani G, et al. Effectiveness of earplugs in preventing recreational noise–induced hearing loss: a randomized clinical trial. JAMA Otolaryngol Head Neck Surg 2016;142(6):551–8.
16. Alemi AS, Chan DK. Progressive hearing loss and head trauma in enlarged vestibular aqueduct: a systematic review and meta-analysis. Otolaryngol Head Neck Surg 2015;153(4):512–7.
17. Hoosein MM, Banerjee AR, Vaidhyanath R. The dilated vestibular aqueduct: a diagnosis not to be missed. J Emerg Med 2012;43(5):e331–2.
18. Kou B, Macdonald R. Toronto's Hospital for Sick Children study of traumatic sudden sensorineural hearing loss. J Otolaryngol 1998;27(2):64–8.
19. Madden C, Halsted M, Benton C, et al. Enlarged vestibular aqueduct syndrome in the pediatric population. Otol Neurotol 2003;24(4):625–32.

Nasal Injuries in Sports

Alexander P. Marston, MD, Erin K. O'Brien, MD,
Grant S. Hamilton III, MD*

KEYWORDS

- Nasal fracture • Septal deviation • Septal fracture • Septal hematoma

KEY POINTS

- In the setting of sports-related trauma, the nasal bones are the most frequently fractured facial bones.
- The goals of nasal fracture treatment are to restore the preinjury nasal appearance and function.
- The ideal timing for nasal fracture reduction is between 3 and 10 days after an injury.
- Untreated septal fractures and deviations are the most common reason for revision nasal reconstructive surgery.

INTRODUCTION

Nasal bone fracture is a commonly encountered injury in individuals participating in both recreational and competitive sports. Of the facial fractures that occur in the setting of sports activities, the nasal bones are the most frequently fractured.[1] Injury to the nose can present along a wide spectrum of severity from limited pain and swelling to obvious traumatic deformity and asymmetry. The evaluating physician is faced with the challenge of appropriate diagnosis, consideration for referral to a specialist, and immediate versus delayed treatment interventions. With the nose being a central feature of facial aesthetics and an important component of the upper respiratory tract, achieving excellent treatment results is critical to maintaining quality of life. The specific goals of nasal fracture treatment are to restore the premorbid nasal form and function. The treatment of nasal bone fractures dates back to the beginning of documented medicine and is reported as early as the fifth century BC when Hippocrates described a multitude of reduction and splinting techniques.[2] The aim of this article is to discuss the epidemiology, relevant anatomy, pathophysiology, evaluation,

Disclosure Statement: G.S. Hamilton has performed consulting work for Spirox, Inc. None of the other authors have any commercial or financial conflicts of interest, and no external funding sources were obtained.
Department of Otorhinolaryngology, Mayo Clinic, 200 1st Street Southwest, Rochester, MN 55905, USA
* Corresponding author.
E-mail address: hamilton.grant@mayo.edu

workup, treatment, potential complications, and convalescence related to traumatic nasal injuries in the setting of sports activities.

EPIDEMIOLOGY

Sports-related injuries and assaults are responsible for most nasal fractures.[3] Young men are most likely to be affected, and the peak incidence occurs between the second and third decades of life.[3] With the nasal pyramid projecting from the midface, it is vulnerable to injury and, therefore, the most common of all facial bone fractures.[4] Specifically in the setting of sports activities, the nasal bones are also at greatest risk of fracture when compared with other facial fractures.[1] In a 2000 survey of 767 facial fractures treated by facial plastics surgeons, 63% were nasal fractures and 49% of these injuries were deemed sports related.[5] In a 2011 study, 91 patients incurred a nasal injury during a sporting activity. Of this group, 65% were diagnosed with nasal bone fractures, 70% were in males and 87% occurred in a noncontact sport.[6] In this cohort, organized rather than recreational competition was the more common setting for sports-related nasal fractures to occur (59% vs 41%). Additionally, it was determined that most nasal injuries happened while playing a noncontact team sport, such as basketball, baseball, soccer, and softball. Only 13.2% of the nasal fractures were the result of a football, traditionally a high-contact sport.

Facial fractures in children younger than 5 years are rare; however, the incidence increases with age. By the time one reaches the 16- to 20-year-old age range, the incidence is nearly twice the total population rate.[7] Perkins and colleagues[5] reported that 42% of all nasal fractures occurred in individuals 17 years of age and younger but that this younger population was responsible for 61% of the sports-related nasal fractures. With increasing age, children typically participate in more competitive and high-speed sports activities leading to a higher risk of sustaining facial trauma in the setting of athletic participation.

ANATOMY

The upper third of the nose is a pyramid-shaped structure often referred to as the bony vault. The paired nasal bones are centrally located with the frontal processes of the maxilla articulating at the lateral surfaces of the nasal bones (**Fig. 1**). The lacrimal and ethmoid bones are deep to the bony vault and help support its projected position. The ethmoid bone contributes to the bony labyrinth of the paranasal sinuses and to the bony nasal septum. The septum is composed of cartilage anteriorly and bone posteriorly. The bony septum consists of the perpendicular plate of the ethmoid bone, vomer, and the nasal crest of the palatine bone and maxilla (**Fig. 2**). The cartilaginous septum is made up of the quadrangular cartilage. Where the septal cartilage abuts the vomer posteriorly and the maxillary crest inferiorly, a bony groove provides stability of the bony-cartilaginous articulation and allows for slight lateral mobility of the septal cartilage.[8] During the compressive forces sustained from nasal trauma, this mobility helps to prevent septal fractures. The middle third of the nose includes the paired upper lateral cartilages, which fuse in the midline with the dorsal surface of the quadrangular septal cartilage. Laterally, the upper lateral cartilages articulate with the frontal processes of the maxillae via the piriform ligaments.[9] The cranial or superior aspect of the upper lateral cartilage overlaps with the nasal bones. This region is termed the *keystone* area and is crucial to recreate when reconstructing severe traumatic nasal deformities. The lower third of the nose contains the lower lateral cartilages. These paired structures are made up of the medial, intermediate, and lateral crura (**Fig. 3**). The major tip support structures

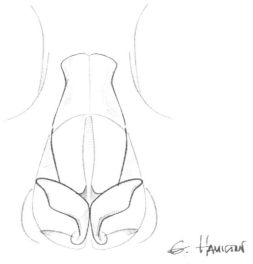

Fig. 1. Coronal image depicting the relationship of the nasal bones, upper and lower lateral cartilages within the upper, middle, and lower thirds of the nose, respectively.

of the nose arise from the lower lateral cartilages. Specifically, tip support is derived from the orientation and resiliency of the lower lateral cartilages, the medial crura attachments to the caudal nasal septum, and the attachment of the lower and upper lateral cartilages.[10] Similar to the *keystone* area of the upper lateral cartilages and

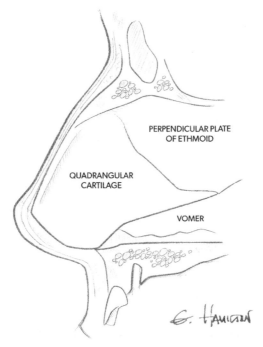

Fig. 2. Sagittal image of the nasal septum showing the perpendicular plate of the ethmoid bone, vomer, nasal crest of the palatine bone and maxilla, and quadrangular cartilage.

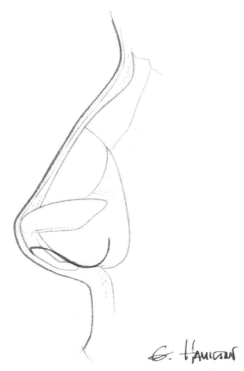

Fig. 3. Sagittal image depicting the relationship of the nasal bones, upper and lower lateral cartilages within the upper, middle and lower thirds of the nose, respectively.

nasal bones, the *scroll* is a supportive structure created by overlap of the upper and lower lateral cartilages.[11] The arterial supply of the nose is derived from both the internal and external carotid arteries systems. The anterior and posterior ethmoid arteries, dorsal nasal artery, and external nasal artery all arise from the ophthalmic artery, a branch of the internal carotid artery. The external carotid artery supplies the nose via branches of the facial and internal maxillary arteries. Specifically, the infraorbital and sphenopalatine arteries arise from the internal maxillary artery and the superior labial and angular arteries arise from the facial artery. The venous drainage travels predominantly through the facial and pterygoid veins into the internal jugular vein or via the ophthalmic vein through the cavernous sinus. Sensation of both the external nasal skin and internal nasal mucosal lining is supplied by the first and second branches of the fifth cranial nerve.

PATHOGENESIS/PATHOPHYSIOLOGY

The patients' age, force sustained, directional impact, and the type of object striking the nose all impact the severity and type of nasal injury sustained. In general, older adults experience fractures that are comminuted because of the inelastic and more demineralized state of the nasal bones.[12] In younger people, dislocation and simple fractures of the nasal bones are more common given the increased elasticity of the cartilage and bony nasal framework. Lateral forces are the more common directional mechanism of injury; however, deviated fractures of the nasal bones can occur in a similar fashion from both lateral and frontal blows to the nose.[13] Nasal injuries can range from simple hematomas and superficial lacerations to complex open nasal and facial bone fractures. The varied types and presentations of nasal fractures make a single severity scale impractical; however, the general description of a nasal fracture can be described as follows:

- Laterality
  - Unilateral versus bilateral
- Fracture type
  - Open versus closed
  - Displaced versus nondisplaced
  - Simple versus comminuted versus greenstick
- Nasal bone fracture position:
  - Deviated from midline
  - Medialized versus lateralized
  - Impacted or telescoped
  - Open book: lateral splay of the nasal bones leading to nasal dorsum widening
- Septal fracture
  - Cartilaginous versus bony septal fracture
- Fractures of adjacent facial structures
  - Orbital rim/floor fractures
  - Nasorbitoethmoidal fracture
  - Midface fracture involving the maxilla or zygoma
  - LeFort-type fracture
  - Mandibular fracture

EVALUATION
History

As with any trauma evaluation, primary consideration should be given to patients' airway, breathing, and circulation. Associated intracranial and cervical spine injuries should be evaluated and the appropriate precautions followed. When taking a history, it is important to ask about the timing of the trauma, nature and direction of the striking object, loss of consciousness, pain, nasal obstruction, altered appearance or new asymmetry of the nose, bloody or clear nasal drainage, diminished sense of smell, vision change, and malocclusion. A thorough examination is critical to accurately assess the type and severity of nasal injury.

Physical Examination

- Basic examination supplies include the following: light source, nasal speculum, Frazier suction device, cotton-tipped applicators.
- Perform a careful evaluation of the appearance of the nose from varying perspectives to assess for ecchymosis, laceration, deviation, flattening, broadening, loss of nasal length.
- Obtain multi-view photographs of the face with respect to the Frankfurt horizontal, when appropriate:
  - Front
  - Right and left oblique
  - Right and left profile
  - Base (looking up to the nose from below the chin)
  - Skyline (looking down on the nose from above the head)
- Palpate the bony vault of the nose to assess for nasal bone step-offs, mobility, and crepitus.

- For anterior rhinoscopy, do the following:
  - Use a light source and nasal speculum for the intranasal examination.
  - Clear blood and secretions with suction.
  - Evaluate for the following:
    - Epistaxis
    - Clear nasal drainage
- The following may indicate a cerebrospinal fluid leak:
  - Compressible blue or red appearing submucosal mass
- The following may indicate a septal hematoma:
  - Septal mucosal lacerations
  - Septal deviation or fracture
- If available, perform rigid or flexible nasal endoscopy for a more detailed intranasal evaluation.

Radiographic Workup

The diagnosis of a nasal bone fracture is most commonly confirmed from the history and physical examination alone. Logan and colleagues[14] investigated 100 consecutive patients who presented to the emergency department with nasal bone fractures and determined that nasal bone radiographs did not significantly change or impact the diagnosis or management of the nasal trauma. However, in some cases, insurance companies will require objective radiographic evidence of nasal bone deviation or fracture before surgical authorization. If an isolated nasal bone fracture is suspected, high-resolution ultrasonography can also be considered. Lee and colleagues[15] reported on 140 consecutive patients with nasal trauma and found that the accuracy rates for high-resolution ultrasound, computed tomography, and conventional radiography to confirm the diagnosis of a nasal fracture to be 100%, 92%, and 79%, respectively. Computed tomography is obtained in cases of complex nasal bone fractures or suspicion of associated facial, orbital, or mandibular fractures.

MANAGEMENT

Acute management of nasal trauma may require laceration repair, control of epistaxis, and/or drainage of a septal hematoma. In patients who have sustained nasal trauma, the goals of treatment are to establish an acceptable nasal appearance by reducing the nasal bones and septum to their premorbid location, achieve bilateral nasal airway patency, preserve external and internal nasal valve structure, and prevent intranasal stenosis or septal perforation.[16] Definitive treatment of a nasal fracture can be completed immediately or in a delayed fashion; however, the most common practice is to reexamine patients 3 to 5 days following the injury to better assess the nose in the setting of reduced edema. The ideal timing for nasal fracture reduction is between 3 and 10 days after the injury. If more than 2 weeks is allowed to elapse, adequate reduction is difficult to achieve because of the deposition of fibrous connective tissue.[3] Nasal fractures ranging from simple to complex can be treated with combined closed nasal bone reduction and endonasal techniques for septal repair. However, in cases of severe deformities, an open septorhinoplasty approach may be indicated for internal fixation and cartilage or bone grafting. In cases of complex nasal fractures, a surgery consultation should be requested to determine if an open or endonasal approach is indicated.

Nasal Laceration Repair

Lacerations on the surface of the nose should be copiously irrigated. Level 1B and 2C evidence demonstrates that irrigation with polyhexanide/betaine or povidone-iodine, respectively, enhances wound healing.[17] For severe cases of nasal trauma, the external skin, cartilage, and intranasal mucosa may all be violated. In this circumstance, it is important to close all 3 layers of injured tissue. Reapproximate lacerated nasal cartilage with an interrupted 5-0 monofilament absorbable suture. Lacerated nasal skin can be sutured in either a vertical mattress or simple interrupted fashion using fine, nonabsorbable monofilament suture. Alternatively, 5-0 fast absorbing surgical gut suture can be used for skin closure if patients do not wish to return for suture removal. Following repair of a nasal cartilage laceration, consider securing a fluoroplastic nasal bolster (0.5-mm thickness) with 3-0 nylon along the internal and external surfaces of the nasal sidewall. Gently tie the bolster in place so as not to compromise the blood supply. The bolster and permanent sutures should be removed after 5 to 7 days.

Septal Hematoma

Identification and drainage of a septal hematoma following injury to the nose is important to minimize postoperative morbidity. The perichondrium adheres tightly to the septal cartilage and provides its blood supply. A septal hematoma occurs between the septal cartilage and perichondrium, effectively separating the cartilage from its nutrient source.[11] If a septal hematoma is not properly drained, pressure-induced avascular necrosis can occur within 3 days.[18] Septal cartilage necrosis is associated with several avoidable complications, including septal abscess, septal perforation, saddle nose deformity, columellar retraction, and nasal base widening.

Septal Hematoma Incision and Drainage

- Equipment includes the following: light source, nasal speculum, Frazier suction device, cotton-tipped applicators, 0.05% oxymetazoline nasal spray, 4% cocaine on nasal pledgets, 1% lidocaine with 1:100,000 epinephrine, 18-Ga needle on a 10-mL syringe, No. 15 blade scalpel, 18-Ga angiocatheter, saline irrigation, small surgical clamp, 0.25-in Penrose drain, 4-0 nylon suture, material to gently compress the septal flaps (Merocel nasal tampon [Medtronic, Minneapolis, MN] Doyle nasal splints, and so forth).
- Suction the nasal cavities free of blood and debris.
- Perform an intranasal examination with nasal speculum and/or flexible fiberoptic nasal endoscope to evaluate for areas of swelling.
  - Septal hematomas have a more blue or reddish hue than the surrounding mucosa.
- Palpate areas of swelling with cotton-tipped applicators.
  - Septal hematomas are compressible.
- Apply nasal decongestant spray, such as 0.05% oxymetazoline or 4% cocaine on nasal pledgets.
  - Septal hematomas do not shrink in size with decongestion.
  - Topical cocaine is safe to use on nasal mucosa. The maximum topical dose is 3 mg/kg. Therefore, for an 80-kg adult, up to 6 mL can safely be used.
- If a septal hematoma is identified, drain immediately.
- Inject 1% lidocaine with 1:100,000 epinephrine for local anesthesia.
  - Injection of epinephrine, a vasoconstrictive agent, is safe to use in the nose despite previously published warnings to avoid this anatomic location.
- Aspirate blood with an 18-Ga needle on a 10-mL syringe to confirm the diagnosis.
- Incise over the drained hematoma with a No. 15 blade.
- Gently spread using a surgical clamp to ensure the hematoma is completely decompressed.

- Irrigate with saline on an 18-Ga angiocatheter.
- Place a 0.25-in Penrose drain into the opened hematoma cavity and suture in place across the nasal septum with a 4-0 nylon suture.
- Place a Merocel or polymeric silicone (Silastic, Dow Corning, Midland, MI) stent on both sides of the septal hematoma to prevent reaccumulation of blood.
- Use an oral antibiotic with broad-spectrum coverage against upper respiratory flora, such as a penicillin-based antibiotic with a beta-lactamase inhibitor or clindamycin.
- There should be an outpatient follow-up in 3 days with an otolaryngologist.

Closed Reduction with Digital Manipulation for Minimally Displaced Nasal Fractures

In patients who experience a closed, minimally displaced nasal fracture, a common result is an isolated deviation or alteration of the nasal bones from their premorbid state. If there is minimal edema and no associated injuries requiring medical attention, an immediate closed reduction with digital manipulation can be attempted. Although each nasal fracture occurs in a unique and unpredictable fashion, lateral force blows can lead to depression or medialization of the ipsilateral nasal bone and lateralization of the contralateral nasal bone. On occasion, the medialized nasal bone is in a more aesthetically favorable location after the injury; therefore, reducing the lateralized bone may be the only treatment necessary. The physician can then discuss with patients about the possibility of closed reduction in which digital pressure will be applied externally to reestablish nasal bone symmetry. Topical cocaine and regional lidocaine injections can be used to anesthetize the nose. Zide and Swift[19] published an excellent primer on regional anesthesia of the face. It is important to communicate with patients that if the reduction generates pain or discomfort, the treatment can be discontinued at the patients' request. With the palmar surface of the examiner's thumb against the lateralized segment of the nasal bone and the fingers extending beyond the malar eminence, broad gentle force is exerted at the site of the bony step-off (**Figs. 4** and **5**). Progressively more pressure is applied until movement of the nasal bone is achieved to the desired position. Often, an audible or palpable click indicates successful repositioning of the nasal bone. The disadvantage of this technique is that the physician has limited control over the nasal bone segments. Consequently, this approach will likely fail when the fragmented segments overlap one another or if the desired result is to lateralize an in-fractured nasal bone. If patients cannot tolerate the manipulation or an unsatisfactory result is achieved, reduction under general anesthesia is then recommended.

Closed Nasal Fracture Reduction Under General Anesthesia

For nasal fractures that involve more severe deviation and comminution or in patients who do not wish to attempt digital reduction as described earlier, treatment in the operating room under general anesthesia is the preferred setting to achieve optimal results.

- General anesthesia is induced with a down RAE endotracheal tube.
- Patients are positioned supine, and the operating table is rotated 180° away from the anesthesia unit.
- Presurgical prep supplies are depicted in **Fig. 6**.
  - Chlorhexidine-based skin prep is used to clean the face.
  - Pledgets soaked in 0.05% oxymetazoline are placed in the nasal cavities.
  - Preoperative nasal markings may be made with a marking pen to denote the sites of nasal bone deviation.

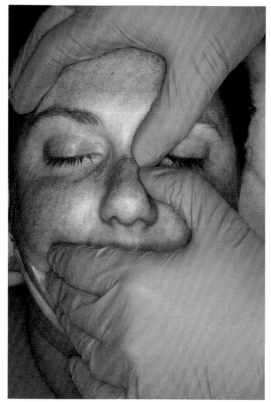

Fig. 4. The thumbs are used to palpate the lateralized segment or step-off of the fractured nasal bone.

- Using a Boies elevator, the external distance from the nostril to a horizontal line passing through the medial canthi is measured (**Fig. 7**).
- The Boies elevator is then grasped with the thumb and forefinger in such a fashion to prevent the instrument from being inserted into the nose beyond the premeasured distance.
  - This step is done to prevent injury to the anterior cranial base.
- First, reduce the medialized or depressed nasal bone using the Boies elevator to apply both anterior and lateral traction on the nasal bone (**Fig. 8**).
- The nondominant hand is placed over the external nasal bone surface to palpate and guide the bone into position.
- After completion of the first reduction maneuver, a potential space is now created to allow the lateralized contralateral nasal bone to be medially repositioned.
- The lateralized nasal bone can be reduced using a combination of external digital manipulation and intranasal stabilization with the Boies elevator.
- When there is concern for instability of free floating nasal bone segments, place a small piece of intranasal absorbable gelatin sponge (Gelfoam, Pfizer Inc, New York, NY) or soft NasoPore (Stryker, Kalamazoo, MI) between the mobile bony segment and the septum. This material need not obstruct the nasal airway or the middle meatus.
- An external nasal splint is applied using a combination of Mastisol (Eloquest Healthcare, Inc, Ferndale, MI), Steri-Strip (3M, St Paul, MN) and Aquaplast.

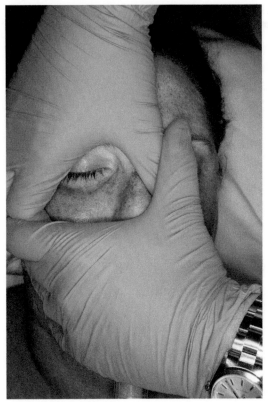

Fig. 5. The fingers are grasped around the contralateral zygoma, and pressure is exerted on the fractured nasal bone in a medial direction. A palpable click is often appreciated when reduction is achieved.

- The nasal splint provides modest protection against reinjury and reminds patients to take precaution not to traumatize the nose. The taping under the splint can also speed resolution of the edema. The splint is kept in place for 7 days.
- Use broad-spectrum postoperative antibiotics for 7 days.

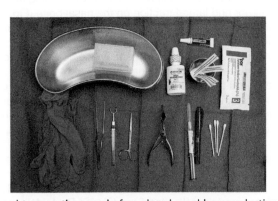

Fig. 6. Supplies used to prep the nose before closed nasal bone reduction.

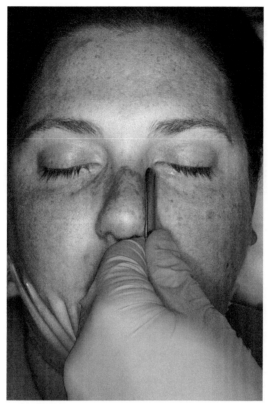

Fig. 7. A Boies elevator is used to approximate the external distance from the nostril to the nasal bone. This step is performed to reduce the risk of injury to the anterior cranial base.

Septal Deviation and Fracture

Traumatic distortion or fracture of the nasal septum commonly occurs in conjunction with nasal bone fractures and is important to address at the time of surgical repair. A deviated or fractured nasal septum can exert tension on the bony nasal pyramid, and complete reduction may be inhibited if a septal injury is not properly repaired. Therefore, the septum should be addressed before nasal bone reduction. Rohrich and Adams[20] reported that the most common reason for unsuccessful nasal bone reduction is failure to properly reduce the nasal septum. The pattern of septal fractures as demonstrated in cadaver studies shows that both lateral and frontal force injuries can produce C-shaped cartilaginous and bony septal fractures.[13,21] Closed reduction of the nasal septum can sometimes be achieved with Asch forceps when the inferior aspect of the septum is disarticulated off of the nasal spine and maxillary crest. In cases of unsuccessful closed reduction or severely comminuted septal fractures, an endonasal septoplasty should be performed via a hemitransfixion incision. For this technique, an incision through the anterior nasoseptal mucosa is fashioned and mucoperichondrial flaps are elevated. This approach allows for improved visualization of the traumatic septal deformity and more precise reduction of the septal fragments. In cases of severe trauma, an open rhinoplasty approach may be necessary.

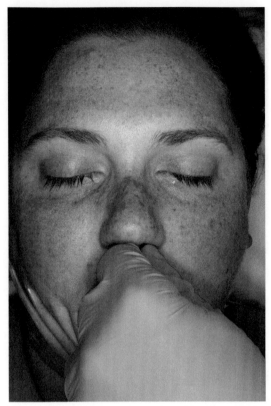

Fig. 8. The Boies elevator is grasped with the thumb and forefinger in such a fashion to prevent the instrument from being inserted into the nose beyond the premeasured distance, and the medialized nasal bone is reduced using both anterior and lateral forces on the Boies elevator.

Pediatric Nasal Trauma

The pediatric nasal structures are more malleable and less prone to comminution than the adult nose because of their higher cartilaginous content. When nasal trauma does occur in children, fractures can be challenging to diagnose because of the rapid development of soft tissue edema and subsequent masking of the underlying deformity. In general, the least invasive treatment option should be performed to correct traumatic pediatric nasal obstruction or deformity.[11] The nasal septum, including the vomer, ethmoid bone, and septal cartilage, serves as a growth center for the nose and midface.[22] Animal studies have demonstrated that removing the septum early in life can lead to restricted nasal development, midface hypoplasia, and malocclusion.[23] However, subsequent animal studies showed that submucous resection of septal cartilage with mucoperichondrial flap preservation did not result in growth disturbances. In clinical pediatric studies, numerous reports have found no significant long-term growth restriction when septoplasty is performed with preservation of the mucoperichondrium. Therefore, closed reduction procedures are now recommended with similar indications as described in the adult population (**Fig. 9**).[24] The one exception to pediatric nasal trauma management is that if an open septorhinoplasty is required, this is delayed until patients' facial skeleton and nose are fully developed. In addition to

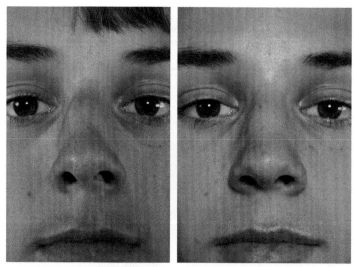

Fig. 9. The image on the left demonstrates a nasal fracture sustained in a 15-year-old boy with rightward deviation of the nasal dorsum following trauma to the nose. The image on the right shows the result achieved after closed reduction of his nasal fracture.

preserving the mucoperichondrium, segments of septal bone and cartilage should be replaced within the injured nose. As a means of organizing the resected septal pieces, polydioxanone foil plates can be used to secure the segments in an ideal orientation before replacement within the reconstructed septum.

Outcomes

When patient satisfaction is used to judge the success of nasal fracture treatment, reports find that between 70% and 90% of patients achieve a successful result.[25–27] However, surgeon and patient perception of success has been shown to differ significantly. Staffel[27] reported on 105 nasal fractures that were treated with either closed or open reduction and found that on follow-up analysis, 79% of patients versus only 39% of surgeons were satisfied with the overall treatment result. Illum[25] reported on 88 patients who had undergone closed nasal fracture reduction and found that 91% of patients were satisfied at 3 months, 87% were satisfied at 3 years and only 3% went on to have an open septorhinoplasty procedure. In general, closed treatment techniques yield acceptable long-term results for mild to moderate severity nasal bone fractures. In children who have nasal trauma, the long-term functional results have been shown to be similar in individuals who sustained a nasal fracture as a child versus normal controls with respect to nasal obstruction, whereas aesthetic variations, such as nasal asymmetries and saddle deformities, were more common in the fracture group.[28] A common pitfall that can lead to inadequate nasal fracture reduction and to the later development of nasal obstruction is failure to completely treat a septal fracture or deviation. Careful attention and treatment of an injured nasal septum should be addressed at the time of primary surgical repair to best avoid secondary reconstructive procedures.

COMPLICATIONS

Table 1 summarizes the most likely complications of the treatment of nasal injuries.

Table 1
Common complications in the treatment of nasal injuries

Complication	Cause	Acute Signs and Symptoms	Long-Term Sequelae
Septal abscess	Undrained septal hematoma	Nasal tip tenderness, pain out of proportion to examination	Septal perforation, saddle nose deformity
Septal necrosis	Potential consequence of untreated septal hematoma or abscess	Nasal tip tenderness, pain out of proportion to examination	Septal perforation, saddle nose deformity, intracranial infection
Cavernous sinus thrombosis	Undrained nasal septal abscess	Lethargy, focal neurologic findings	Meningitis, brain abscess, sepsis
Cerebrospinal fluid leak	Injury to the anterior cranial base	Clear nasal drainage, salty or metallic taste	Intracranial infection
Lacrimal duct obstruction	Injury to the nasolacrimal duct system	Epiphora	Epiphora
Sinusitis	Untreated septal deviation causing ostiomeatal complex obstruction	Nasal obstruction, facial pain, purulent nasal drainage	Chronic rhinosinusitis, mucocele, anosmia
Toxic shock syndrome	Retained nasal pack after reduction, failure to provide antistaphylococcal antibiotics	Nasal pain, purulent drainage	Intracranial infection, sepsis
Untreated nasorbitoethmoidal fracture	Complex facial and nasal trauma; injury to the medial canthal ligament	Increased intercanthal distance (>35 mm), telescoped nasal bones, blunting of the medial canthus	Widened nasal dorsum, alteration of facial appearance

RETURN TO SPORT PARTICIPATION

Although the fractured nasal bone segments may be mobile for approximately 2 weeks after reduction, it is recommended to wait between 6 and 8 weeks before returning to competitive sports participation. The presence of a recent nasal fracture causes no specific problem to playing a sport; however, there is significant risk of reinjury in the setting of premature physical activity. When return to sports play cannot be postponed, protective facial masks should be worn and may help prevent a subsequent fracture (**Fig. 10**).[29] Regardless of the time spent away from playing sports, nearly all athletes are able to return to their premorbid level of sports participation.[6]

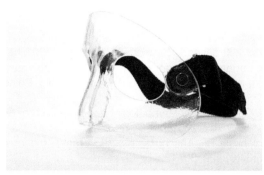

Fig. 10. A custom midface mask can help prevent reinjury when returning to contact sports. (Graphica Medica, Bloomington, MN.)

SUMMARY

- Complex nasal lacerations must be repaired in 3 separate layers, including the nasal mucosa, cartilage, and external skin.
- The nasal bones are the most frequently fractured facial bones in the setting of sports-related trauma.
- Most nasal injuries occur while playing a noncontact team sport.
- Important historical parameters in determining the type and severity of a nasal injury include the force sustained, directional impact, and the type of object striking the nose.
- The goals of nasal fracture treatment are to restore the preinjury nasal appearance and function.
- Acute management of a nasal fracture may require control of epistaxis and/or drainage of a septal hematoma.
- Older adults generally experience fractures that are comminuted due to the inelastic and more demineralized state of the nasal bones
- The ideal timing for nasal fracture reduction is between 3 and 10 days after the injury. Repair before 2 weeks is preferred to minimize the effects of newly deposited scar and fibrous tissue.
- Untreated septal fractures and deviations are the most common reason for revision surgery; therefore, it is important to properly address septal injuries at the time of the primary reconstructive procedure.
- Closed reduction with digital manipulation or endonasal repositioning techniques can be used for mild to moderate severity nasal bone fracture deformities.
- Severe, complex nasal trauma requires an open septorhinoplasty approach.
- Pediatric nasal trauma can be safely addressed and treated in a similar fashion as adult nasal trauma; however, open reconstructive procedures should be delayed until the facial skeleton and nose are completely developed.
- If a septoplasty is required in a child, maintain and replace as much cartilage and bone in the septum as possible.
- Long-term patient satisfaction is reported to be between 70% and 90% following closed treatment of nasal bone fractures.
- Return to sports participation is typically delayed for 6 to 8 weeks after sustaining a nasal bone fracture. A protective nasal mask should be worn if sports participation occurs before 6 to 8 weeks.

REFERENCES

1. Frenguelli A, Ruscito P, Bicciolo G, et al. Head and neck trauma in sporting activities. Review of 208 cases. J Craniomaxillofac Surg 1991;19(4):178–81.
2. Lascaratos JG, Segas JV, Trompoukis CC, et al. From the roots of rhinology: the reconstruction of nasal injuries by Hippocrates. Ann Otol Rhinol Laryngol 2003; 112(2):159–62.
3. Cummings CW. Cummings otolaryngology head & neck surgery. 4th edition. Philadelphia: Elsevier Mosby; 2005.
4. Friese G, Wojciehoski RF. The nose: bleeds, breaks and obstructions. Emerg Med Serv 2005;34(8):129–30, 132–5, 137.
5. Perkins SW, Dayan SH, Sklarew EC, et al. The incidence of sports-related facial trauma in children. Ear Nose Throat J 2000;79(8):632–4, 636, 638.
6. Cannon CR, Cannon R, Young K, et al. Characteristics of nasal injuries incurred during sports activities: analysis of 91 patients. Ear Nose Throat J 2011;90(8): E8–12.
7. Azevedo AB, Trent RB, Ellis A. Population-based analysis of 10,766 hospitalizations for mandibular fractures in California, 1991 to 1993. J Trauma 1998;45(6): 1084–7.
8. Pitanguy I. Revisiting the dermocartilaginous ligament. Plast Reconstr Surg 2001; 107(1):264–6.
9. Craig JR, Bied A, Landas S, et al. Anatomy of the upper lateral cartilage along the lateral pyriform aperture. Plast Reconstr Surg 2015;135(2):406–11.
10. Pasha R. Otolaryngology: head & neck surgery: clinical reference guide. 2nd edition. San Diego (CA): Plural Pub; 2006.
11. Olsen KD, Carpenter RJ 3rd, Kern EB. Nasal septal trauma in children. Pediatrics 1979;64(1):32–5.
12. Colton JJ, Beekhuis GJ. Management of nasal fractures. Otolaryngol Clin North Am 1986;19(1):73–85.
13. Harrison DH. Nasal injuries: their pathogenesis and treatment. Br J Plast Surg 1979;32(1):57–64.
14. Logan M, O'Driscoll K, Masterson J. The utility of nasal bone radiographs in nasal trauma. Clin Radiol 1994;49(3):192–4.
15. Lee MH, Cha JG, Hong HS, et al. Comparison of high-resolution ultrasonography and computed tomography in the diagnosis of nasal fractures. J Ultrasound Med 2009;28(6):717–23.
16. Bailey BJ. Head and neck surgery–otolaryngology. 3rd edition. Philadelphia: Lippincott Williams & Wilkins; 2001.
17. Wilkins RG, Unverdorben M. Wound cleaning and wound healing: a concise review. Adv Skin Wound Care 2013;26(4):160–3.
18. Fry HJ. The pathology and treatment of haematoma of the nasal septum. Br J Plast Surg 1969;22(4):331–5.
19. Zide BM, Swift R. How to block and tackle the face. Plast Reconstr Surg 1998; 101(3):840–51.
20. Rohrich RJ, Adams WP Jr. Nasal fracture management: minimizing secondary nasal deformities. Plast Reconstr Surg 2000;106(2):266–73.
21. Murray JA, Maran AG, Mackenzie IJ, et al. Open v closed reduction of the fractured nose. Arch Otolaryngol 1984;110(12):797–802.
22. Ousterhout DK, Vargervik K. Maxillary hypoplasia secondary to midfacial trauma in childhood. Plast Reconstr Surg 1987;80(4):491–9.

23. Sarnat BG, Wexler MR. Longitudinal development of upper facial deformity after septal resection in growing rabbits. Br J Plast Surg 1969;22(4):313–23.

24. Lawrence R. Pediatric septoplasy: a review of the literature. Int J Pediatr Otorhinolaryngol 2012;76(8):1078–81.

25. Illum P. Long-term results after treatment of nasal fractures. J Laryngol Otol 1986; 100(3):273–7.

26. Crowther JA, O'Donoghue GM. The broken nose: does familiarity breed neglect? Ann R Coll Surg Engl 1987;69(6):259–60.

27. Staffel JG. Optimizing treatment of nasal fractures. Laryngoscope 2002;112(10): 1709–19.

28. Grymer LF, Gutierrez C, Stoksted P. Nasal fractures in children: influence on the development of the nose. J Laryngol Otol 1985;99(8):735–9.

29. Morita R, Shimada K, Kawakami S. Facial protection masks after fracture treatment of the nasal bone to prevent re-injury in contact sports. J Craniofac Surg 2007;18(1):143–5.

Maxillofacial and Mandibular Fractures in Sports

Christopher F. Viozzi, DDS, MD

KEYWORDS

- Mandibular fracture • Maxillary fracture • Zygoma fracture • Orbital fracture

KEY POINTS

- Sports activities account for between 3% and 29% of facial injuries and 10% and 42% of facial fractures depending on the population under study.
- Mandibular fractures can cause acute airway compromise in athletes owing to severe bleeding as well as posterior displacement of the muscles that support airway patency.
- Zygoma fractures can result in significant ocular problems both in the acute setting and over the longer term.
- The most common fractures of the facial skeleton related to sports activities are nasal, mandibular, and zygoma fractures.
- Decisions regarding return to play must be individualized, considering age, compliance, pattern of injury, treatment, time since injury, and the likelihood of another facial injury.

INTRODUCTION

Various studies have evaluated the extent to which athletic injuries contribute to the overall incidence of facial fractures. In 1 review, sports accounted for between 3% and 29% of all facial injuries and between 10% and 42% of all facial fractures.[1] In the United States and all developed Western cultures, fractures of the facial skeleton most commonly occur owing to interpersonal violence or motor vehicle crashes. The incidence of facial fractures from sporting activities has clearly decreased over time owing to better preventive measures (helmets, visors, safety glasses, etc). However, this decreasing trend is offset to a certain degree by the emergence of relatively new, more dangerous sports activities, or "pushing the envelope" of traditional sports activities.[2–6] Fractures can occur from contact between athletes, and between athletes and their surroundings (including their equipment). Contact between athletes is the most common cause of facial fractures associated with sporting activities.[7] Football, soccer, hockey, and baseball are involved most frequently in sports-related cases of facial bone fracture, owing to the contact nature of these sports and the high energies sustained during impacts.[1,2,6,7]

Mayo Clinic, 200 First Street Southwest, Rochester, MN 55905, USA
E-mail address: viozzi.christopher@mayo.edu

Clin Sports Med 36 (2017) 355–368
http://dx.doi.org/10.1016/j.csm.2016.11.007
0278-5919/17/© 2016 Elsevier Inc. All rights reserved.

sportsmed.theclinics.com

The force needed to fracture the facial skeleton is actually quite high (**Fig. 1**). The facial skeleton acts as a "crumple zone" to protect the intracranial contents from injury. This undoubtedly evolved as a protective mechanism over millennia. The facial skeleton contains several bony buttresses of thick bone, with intervening thinner bone between (**Fig. 2**). Inside of this lattice are the paranasal sinuses, which serve many functions, including phonation and humidification, as well as a means to lighten the head overall. The practical effect of this arrangement is to disperse and direct energy applied to the anterior and inferior facial region away from the cranium.

Patient age has a significant impact on both the types of injuries that occur and the treatments that can be offered. Growth and development of the face occurs in female patients up to approximately 13 to 16 years of age, with male patients completing facial skeletal growth at approximately 16 to 20 years of age, and occasionally later. The face develops as an inferior-anterior projection of the skull base, assuming an ever-greater presence in the overall head, neck, and cranial anatomy over time. In addition, younger patients tend to have much softer, less calcified bony structures. The combination of these 2 factors means that younger patients have a less prominent face that is more elastic than adult patients, whose facial bones are both less pliable and more prominent. This impacts fracture patterns and incidence accordingly.

The diagnosis of maxillofacial fractures is accomplished via history, including mechanism of injury, combined with physical examination and imaging. The head and neck is a highly vascular and well-innervated region of the body. Therefore, most patients with maxillofacial fractures have severe immediate pain and quickly develop significant

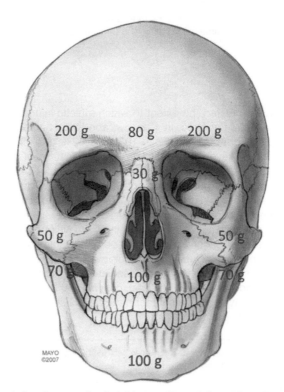

Fig. 1. Forces needed to fracture the facial bones. (Copyright © Mayo Foundation for Medical Education and Research. All rights reserved.)

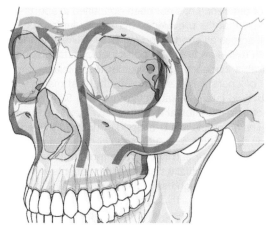

Fig. 2. Horizontal and vertical facial buttresses. (Copyright by AO Foundation, Switzerland. Source: AO Surgery Reference, www.aosurgery.org.)

soft tissue edema over the fractured bones, making clinical examination at best difficult. In addition, the complexity of the facial bony anatomy presents challenges. Some facial fractures with minimal displacement may actually lead to significant morbidity and eventual deformity, yet be difficult to diagnose clinically. Because of this, computed tomography (CT) imaging of patients with suspected maxillofacial fractures has become routine and is available in most hospitals and clinics.

General treatment goals for patients with facial fractures include:

- Identification and treatment of other commonly associated injuries such as closed-head injury, injuries to special sense organs (particularly ocular and auditory systems), and cervical spine injury.
- Restoration of pretraumatic bony anatomy.
- Appropriate support of facial soft tissues and eventual good esthetic outcome.
- Avoidance of facial scarring from either associated soft tissue injuries or from access incisions required to repair the fractures.
- Avoidance of growth disturbance in the growing patient, either from the injury or from the intervention.

The scope of treatments is quite broad, much like other orthopedic treatments. Each patient's injury pattern is unique in some way and, therefore, the specific treatment(s) rendered vary greatly. Some fractures, especially in the young patient, are managed very conservatively via observation and diet restriction, or perhaps a short period of immobilization. Fractures with displacement are generally approached via open reduction procedures, with or without rigid internal fixation.

MANDIBULAR FRACTURES

Fractures of the mandible are among the most common fractures of the facial skeleton.[8] The epidemiology of these injuries varies across cultures and across locations within a specific culture. For example, the patterns of injury seen in the United States is very different in urban areas, where interpersonal violence is the most common cause, and rural areas where motor vehicle collisions are most frequently causative. No matter the culture or the location, studies have consistently shown young male patients tend to be disproportionately more affected than female patients or older patients.[4,6]

Although the gender difference has not been quantified in sports-specific mandibular injuries, it seems likely that the prevalence of mandibular fractures is similar in males and females overall across all sports, and certainly is likely to be similar in sports activities in which both males and females participate.[3] In mandibular fractures caused by sports, the available evidence suggests that these injuries are severe enough to require some form of operative intervention in the vast majority of cases, including open reduction with rigid internal fixation in more than 50% of patients.[9]

Among facial fractures, mandibular fractures have perhaps the highest overall initial risk to the athlete. The mandible is a U-shaped structure that frequently fractures in 2 locations rather than 1, creating a multipiece lower jaw. Because of the proximity to the cranium, coexisting closed-head injury is common. Advanced Cardiac Life Support protocols, when followed, will initially stabilize such patients with cervical spine immobilization on a backboard. Although this is classic Advanced Cardiac Life Support protocol, it may not serve the patient with a significant mandibular fracture well. Mandibular fractures are rarely closed fractures, and tend to bleed significantly from lacerated overlying oral mucosa. The airway itself depends on having an intact mandible, where the insertion of the genioglossus, geniohyoid, and mylohyoid muscles are present and in their appropriate locations (**Fig. 3**). Mandibular fractures, and in particular multipiece fractures permit posterior displacement of these muscle origins, and airway loss can occur, particularly in an obtunded patient. There is a classic aphorism that states, "if you leave the patient facing heaven, it won't be long before they get there," and this rings true in the initial management of patients with mandibular fractures.

Therefore, the initial management begins with ensuring airway patency and the ability of the patient to maintain it. In athletes, this determination is easier, because they are unlikely to be obtunded. Bleeding is self-limiting in most cases, but responds to simple measures such as closing the mouth and biting on gauze. Many mandibular fractures tend to be favorable in terms of their orientation, because muscle activity in the masseter, and the temporalis and medial pterygoids, and the soft tissue envelope tends to reduce these fractures back toward their pretrauma anatomic positions. The natural splinting tendency is to close the mouth, and this helps to stabilize the fractures. Associated dental injuries are very common and lead to more severe bleeding. This topic is covered elsewhere, but mentioned here to emphasize the frequency of this associated problem.

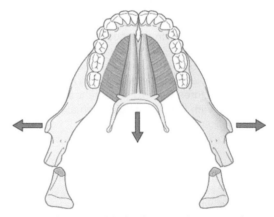

Fig. 3. Airway compromise from mandibular fracture. (*From* Booth PW, Eppley B, Schmelzeisen R. Maxillofacial Trauma and Esthetic Facial Reconstruction. 2011. 2nd edition. Elsevier: Philadelphia; with permission.)

The mandible tends to break in a variety of locations (**Fig. 4**), and in a variety of patterns (frequently in 2 locations, **Fig. 5**). Therefore, the signs and symptoms vary widely. A common pattern is a mandibular angle fracture on 1 side, with a contralateral fracture of the condylar process. Classic signs of acute mandibular fracture are listed in **Box 1**.

The definitive diagnosis is via plain film imaging sometimes supplemented by CT. An orthopantomogram (panorex, panellipse) radiograph (**Fig. 6**) is available in most hospital emergency departments and is the initial radiograph of choice for any patient with suspected mandibular bony injury. This radiograph is often enough to permit not only definitive diagnosis, but also definitive treatment. Radiation dosage from this image is orders of magnitude lower than CT, and this consideration is of importance particularly in young patients.

CT can be either used alone, or to supplement plain film imaging. This is particularly true of fractures in the mandibular ramus and condylar process, because these fractures can have more variable degrees of displacement, and the findings on CT imaging can have significant implications regarding definitive management (**Fig. 7**). In addition, many patients with mandibular fracture will be evaluated for closed head injuries with CT imaging. Adding the maxillofacial structures to the head CT is logistically simple and does not require a great deal of time. Obviously, considerations regarding radiation exposure should be balanced against the convenience of simply obtaining CT imaging on every suspected facial fracture. MRI is of very limited use, with the exception of patients with injuries to the soft tissue structures around the temporomandibular joint, where MRI is ideal to determine injuries to the articular cartilage and associated ligamentous structures.

Definitive management of mandibular fractures depends on many factors, including the pattern of fracture(s), and patient factors including comorbidities, other maxillofacial injuries, age, and anticipated compliance. The spectrum of possible treatments includes, from least to most invasive:

- Observation with dietary and functional restrictions;
- Closed "reduction" followed by immobilization with various forms of fixation between the fractured mandible and nonfractured maxilla (intermaxillary fixation, **Fig. 8**);
- Open reduction followed by immobilization;
- Open reduction with rigid or nonrigid internal fixation (via various transoral and/or transcutaneous approaches); and
- Application of external fixators.

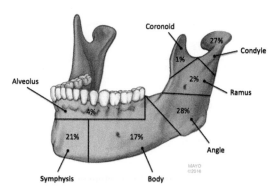

Fig. 4. Anatomic distribution of mandibular fractures. (Copyright © Mayo Foundation for Medical Education and Research. All rights reserved.)

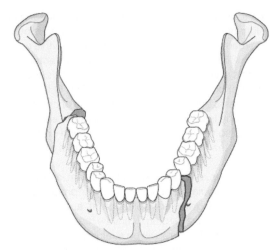

Fig. 5. Bilateral mandibular fracture pattern. (Copyright by AO Foundation, Switzerland. Source: AO Surgery Reference, www.aosurgery.org.)

In general, fractures that are within the ramus or condylar process tend to be treated with immobilization (with or without open reduction). This is a consequence of several factors. Surgical access to this region is impeded by the presence of the facial nerve branches. Even in the best of circumstances, some degree of postoperative dysfunction can occur, and possibly result in permanent facial motor weakness (eg, eyebrow elevation, eyelid closure, elevation of corner of mouth during smiling, puckering). Immobilization time can vary from a few days in younger patients with favorable fractures to 4 weeks or more for ramus fractures with comminution. After release of immobilization, physiotherapy is needed to regain range of motion and rehabilitate atrophied muscles of mastication.

Fractures of the mandibular angle, body, and symphysis (chin) are managed most frequently by open reduction with either rigid or nonrigid internal fixation. This can usually be accomplished via transoral access techniques, thereby eliminating the potential for facial scarring owing to access incisions on the skin. The presence of either developing (in patients under 12 years of age) or erupted teeth complicates the placement of internal fixation devices. Titanium or titanium alloy plate and screw fixation is

---

Box 1
Classic signs of mandibular fracture

- Pain, particularly with motion of the jaw
- Trismus
- Bleeding from lacerated mucosal tissues
- Displaced teeth
- Subjective (or obvious) altered bite
- Palpable or visible "step" in the dental arch
- Bruising or hematoma of the skin overlying the fracture or the sublingual space
- Numbness of the lip or chin owing to injury of the inferior alveolar nerve or its branches

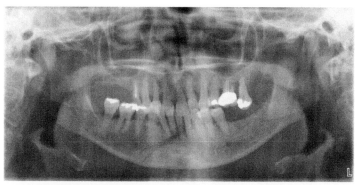

Fig. 6. Panorex film showing bilateral mandibular fracture. Oblique body fracture on the patient's right and subcondylar fracture on patient's left.

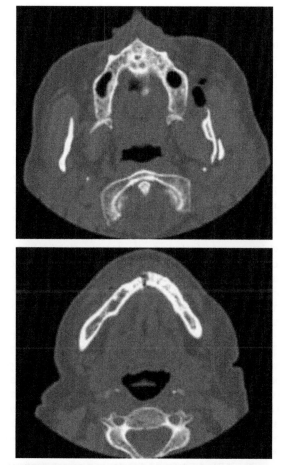

Fig. 7. Computed tomography scan of patient above (panorex shown) showing lateral displacement of proximal left condylar segment, and displacement of anterior body fracture.

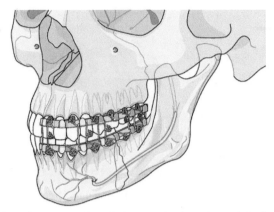

Fig. 8. Intermaxillary fixation with arch bars and wires. (Copyright by AO Foundation, Switzerland. Source: AO Surgery Reference, www.aosurgery.org.)

well-tolerated, biocompatible, and does not obviate the potential for future MRI examinations. The total mass of metal used in facial fracture repair does not typically activate metal detection devices for those who travel frequently.

Major complications from mandibular fractures or their treatment are thankfully rare.[8,10,11] Infections can occur owing to the open nature of these injuries, as well as from injuries to teeth (which can become devitalized and infected from the fracture or the treatment). Fractures that cross the roots of teeth can disrupt the tooth blood supply, leading to pulpal necrosis and abscess. Infected fractures can result in osteomyelitis, but the robust vasculature in the head and neck region makes this a rare problem. More frequently, infections lead to nonunion requiring operative intervention.

Malocclusion is the most common complication of repair, regardless of treatment rendered (even observation). If one considers the exquisite proprioceptive capacity of the dentition, this is not surprising. Minor occlusal abnormalities can be treated with tooth adjustment by the patient's dentist, or possibly via orthodontic tooth movement. Major malocclusion can occur, particularly with fractures of the mandibular condylar process, or in multisegment mandibular fractures. These cases are generally managed with revision surgery, including osteotomies, mobilization of the fracture(s), reduction into proper anatomic alignment, application of reconstruction plates, and possibly bone grafting (autologous or allogeneic).

Injury to sensory nerves is virtually certain from fractures of the mandibular angle, body, and symphysis. All varieties of injury, from stretch injury through transection, can occur.[12] Most often the nerve is not transected, and return of some degree of sensation occurs over 3 to 12 months. Development of pain (dysesthesia) can occur but is rare, and generally managed medically. Transection injuries are indicated for operative repair when they are noted at the time of fracture management.[13] Motor nerve injuries to branches of the facial nerve most frequently occur as a result of operative intervention via transcutaneous approaches. The temporal and marginal mandibular branches are affected most frequently.[14] Partial or complete functional recovery in the nerve and the structures innervated is the rule more than the exception.

As with other fractures, initial bony healing will occur in the first 4 to 6 weeks after injury. This time frame is shortened significantly in the pediatric patient, where initial bony callus formation can occur within 10 to 14 days, and prolonged immobilization can actually lead to fibroosseous or osseous ankylosis of the temporomandibular joint. The opposite is also true; older patients require longer periods of time for primary bony stability to occur.

The question of return to sports activities is invariably important to the athlete with a facial fracture. Although there is no "one size fits all" approach, the author would permit a return to conditioning exercises (aerobic activities and strength training) after 10 to 14 days, so long as the athlete is no longer taking any opioid medications, and assuming they are able to avoid any activities that might cause displacement of the repaired or treated fracture. Obviously, such activities would include any contact sports that carry potential for a blow to the face. In addition, conditioning and strengthening exercises can sometimes cause athletes to "clench" their teeth together, and this can be problematic, depending on the injury and any treatment rendered.

Return to activities that carry a risk of a blow to the face should be delayed an absolute minimum of 8 weeks (preferably 12 weeks) particularly in sports where such a blow would typically be a high-energy contact (football, soccer, hockey). Some of these athletes wear protective headgear that covers the area of fracture (eg, a football helmet in a condylar process injury), or can be modified to do so (baseball/softball helmets, for instance, with a mandibular body fracture).[5] An additional helpful intervention is to have the patient's dentist fabricate a custom mouth guard that will stabilize the mandibular teeth against the maxillary teeth. Use of such a custom guard will help to distribute energy throughout the facial skeletal buttresses in the event of another blow to the mandible.

There are several potential pitfalls for the sports medicine provider involved in the care of patients with mandibular trauma or injury. Perhaps most crucial is the issue of airway management in the acute setting, as discussed. There are situations, however, where a blow to the face causes a mandibular fracture but symptoms may be less than severe, or the athlete continues their activities unaware of a severe injury. Failure to appreciate the potential that an underlying mandibular fracture exists is very real, particularly so in ramus and condylar process fractures, where the only issues may be some arthralgia in the temporomandibular joint region or a minor occlusal disturbance. Delays in care for mandibular fractures, particularly open fractures of the mandibular body or angle increase the potential for infection and nonunion. Delays beyond 7 to 10 days in patients younger than 5 to 7 years of age, beyond 10 to 14 days in patients 8 to 13 years of age, and beyond 14 days in patients up to approximately age 18 years of age raise the potential that initial bony healing may have already occurred, and definitive treatment may require osteotomy of the fractured mandible before reduction and fixation. Finally, because there are no formal guidelines, decisions regarding return to sports activities must be individualized to each patient, considering patient age, compliance, pattern of injury, type of treatment rendered, time since injury, and the likelihood of another facial injury.

Communication with the treating surgeon is important, particularly to understand the potential for problems should such a repeat injury occur early on in the healing phase.[2] Finally, the issue of psychological confidence to return to active participation cannot be understated, not only as regards athletic performance, but also as regards safety. This factor may be more problematic in certain sports than others. For instance, football has facial contact on most plays, baseball the potential for contact with each pitch to a batter, and sports like soccer or lacrosse a less likely occurrence of another facial contact injury. Consultation with a sports psychologist may be warranted in select cases.

MAXILLOFACIAL FRACTURES

The maxillofacial region of the face is generally considered to include the entire face exclusive of the lower facial third (mandible). The large bones that make up this region include the frontal bone and the paired zygoma and maxillary bones. Smaller bones include the nasal, lacrimal, ethmoid, palatine, and portions of the sphenoid bone (**Fig. 9**). This part of the face is termed the midface for obvious reasons, and that term will be used preferentially in this section. For the purposes of this section, the focus is on fractures of the maxilla and zygoma, because orbital and nasal injuries are described elsewhere in detail, albeit with some unavoidable informational overlap with this section. Frontal sinus injuries exist in an area between the face and cranium, and are termed craniofacial fractures, and therefore also not discussed here.

The epidemiology of midface fractures, similar to mandibular fractures, commonly shows younger males as more frequently suffering from these injuries. Specific to athletics, most retrospective reviews show fractures of the zygoma as either most common or second to mandibular fractures in incidence.[2–4,6] Isolated maxillary fractures are actually relatively uncommon in general, and this is also true in athletic injuries. The maxilla is in the middle of many other structures that tend to protect it from injury (crumple zone concept), including the mandible, zygomas, and nasal bones. Therefore, the athlete with a maxillary fracture should be viewed as potentially having other severe injuries, including other facial fractures, closed head injury, and cervical spine injury.

Maxillary fractures have initial airway risk similar in some ways to mandibular fractures. The potential for severe bleeding is actually greater in maxillary fractures, and the pharyngeal constrictor and palatal muscles have attachment points on the maxilla itself. Posterior and inferior displacement of the maxilla (along the skull base) can result in airway compromise. This would be uncommon in all but the most severe athletic injury. The zygoma, in contrast, does not support the airway, but forms a large portion of the bony orbit. Therefore, injury can disrupt the intraocular contents, causing bleeding around and behind the eye. Although not a threat to the airway, such bleeding can be a threat to the patient's vision as a result of problems such as retrobulbar hemorrhage.

The initial management of the patient with a midface fracture includes maintenance of a patent airway, and control of hemorrhage via pressure and elevation of the head if possible. The signs and symptoms of maxillary and zygoma fractures are listed in **Boxes 2** and **3** respectively.

The definitive diagnosis of midface fractures is via CT. Plain film imaging does not play a significant role in evaluating these injuries. As with mandibular fractures, patients with midface fractures can have concomitant head injuries, and CT imaging of

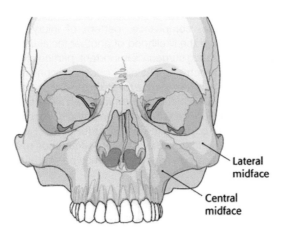

Lateral midface

Central midface

Fig. 9. Bones of the midface (maxillofacial region). (Copyright by AO Foundation, Switzerland. Source: AO Surgery Reference, www.aosurgery.org.)

Box 2
Signs and symptoms of maxillary fracture

- Pain with jaw motion
- Bleeding from lacerated oral mucosa
- Epistaxis
- Displaced teeth
- Alteration in bite (occlusal change)
- Elongation of the face as the midface is displaced backward and inferiorly
- Paresthesia in the distribution of the infraorbital nerve (upper lip, lower eyelid, lateral nose, infraorbital cheek)

---

the head is often a necessary part of the evaluation. In addition, evaluation of the intraorbital contents in cases of zygoma fractures is aided by detailed orbital CT imaging to rule out globe injury and retrobulbar hemorrhage. CT imaging of maxillary fractures will give much more information regarding the degree of comminution and displacement of these bones. Maxillary fractures tend to occur in 3 distinct patterns, classified as Lefort I level, Lefort II level, and Lefort III level, named after the French anatomist Rene Lefort (**Fig. 10**).

Patients with midface fractures should always be evaluated by an ophthalmologist, because studies have shown consistently high risks of ocular injury.[15–17] Midface fractures are nearly always treated in a delayed manner to allow for resolution of edema, thus affording the time to evaluate and manage any ocular injuries.

Definitive management of both maxillary and zygoma fractures depends on the pattern of injury including degree of displacement, presence of other facial fractures, age, and degree of cooperation anticipated. Some zygoma and maxillary fractures are nondisplaced or minimally displaced. This is owing to the "crumple zone effect," wherein the energy from a midface blow is propagated and distributed through the midface bones, dispersing energy with multiple small fractures. This is now an extremely common midface fracture pattern in motor vehicle accidents with airbag deployment, and easily managed with observation, soft diet, pain control, and avoidance of any activities that might further displace the bones involved.

Fractures of the maxilla and zygoma with displacement are managed via open reduction and internal fixation via multiple approaches. Maxillary and zygoma

---

Box 3
Zygoma fracture signs and symptoms

- Pain over the cheekbone
- Depression of the cheekbone with malar flattening or loss of zygomatic arch projection
- Infraorbital nerve paresthesia
- Palpable step in the infraorbital rim
- Diplopia, orbital dystopia, enophthalmous, proptosis
- Extraocular muscle movement abnormalities
- Periorbital and maxillary vestibular ecchymosis and edema
- Subconjunctival hemorrhage

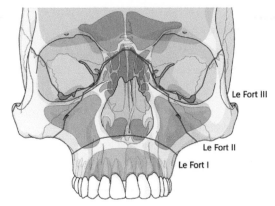

Fig. 10. Maxillary fracture patterns of Lefort I, II, and III. (Copyright by AO Foundation, Switzerland. Source: AO Surgery Reference, www.aosurgery.org.)

fractures are accessed via combinations of intraoral sublabial, eyelid, and coronal incisions depending on the amount of access necessary. Thankfully, these incisions can be made in a manner that is minimally disruptive of facial esthetics. Specific to maxillary fractures, the patient's occlusion needs to be reconstructed by positioning the fractured midface to its appropriate location. This positioning is done via placement of some form of intermaxillary fixation during surgery. Reduction followed by plate and screw fixation is then accomplished. Zygoma fractures involve the orbit by definition, and therefore access to the internal aspects of the bony orbit, including the lateral, inferior (floor), and medial walls is necessary. Once these structures are visualized, reduction and stabilization can proceed.

Over the last decade, the emergence of 3-dimensional radiographic imaging, creation of 3-dimensional anatomic models, intraoperative navigation, and intraoperative CT scanning have all aided surgeons in the management of maxillofacial fractures. A discussion of these modalities is beyond the scope of this article.

Complications in midface fracture repair are specific to each type of fracture. In maxillary fractures, the most common complication is malocclusion, which may require orthognathic jaw surgery for correction. In some cases, orthodontic treatment may suffice. More severe complications include persistent infraorbital nerve paresthesia or dysesthesia, maxillary or ethmoid sinus dysfunction, and lacrimal duct dysfunction with epiphora. These complications are relatively rare and most frequently easily addressed. Zygoma fractures, in contrast, carry significant potential for complications that are severe. From a patient perspective, esthetic deformity from improper reduction to pretrauma anatomy can be very concerning. Late repair (after initial bony healing) of this problem is difficult, and performed via orbitozygomatic osteotomy. Persistent eye problems, such as diplopia, enophthalmous, vertical dystopia, and visual loss, are all potential outcomes of treatment of zygoma fractures and carry significant long-term morbidity for patients.[18]

Return to sports activities after midface fractures would be similar to the discussion points for mandibular fractures. The presence of any associated ocular injury may extend the recommended time needed for appropriate recovery and return to activities. The particular sport in question would also clearly play a role. Collaboration with the patient's ophthalmology provider is essential before returning the athlete to their activities.

Potential pitfalls for the sports medicine provider occur primarily in the acute phase of injury and then at the decision point regarding return to activities. The initial recognition of zygoma and maxillary fractures can be challenging in cases where a low-energy or moderate-energy injury creates fractures that are subtle. Depending on the location of the fracture, particularly in zygoma fractures involving the orbit, failure to appreciate the potential for ocular injury could risk visual disturbance or loss. As with mandibular fractures, there are no formal guidelines regarding return to sports activities, so such decisions must be individualized based on the injuries, type of treatment, time since injury, and the sport involved regarding the potential for another facial injury. Communication with the patient's other providers is key.

REFERENCES

1. Romeo SJ, Hawley CJ, Romeo MW, et al. Facial injuries in sports: a team physician's guide to diagnosis and treatment. Phys Sportsmed 2005;33(4):45–53.
2. Reehal P. Facial injury in sport. Curr Sports Med Rep 2010;9(1):27–34.
3. Murphy C, O'Connell JE, Kearns G, et al. Sports-related maxillofacial injuries. J Craniofac Surg 2015;26(7):2120–3.
4. Montovani JC, de Campos LM, Gomes MA, et al. Etiology and incidence facial fractures in children and adults. Braz J Otorhinolaryngol 2006;72(2):235–41.
5. Laskin DM. Protecting the faces of America. J Oral Maxillofac Surg 2000; 58(4):363.
6. Brook IM, Wood N. Aetiology and incidence of facial fractures in adults. Int J Oral Surg 1983;12(5):293–8.
7. Hwang K, You SH, Lee HS. Outcome analysis of sports-related multiple facial fractures. J Craniofac Surg 2009;20(3):825–9.
8. Ramadhan A, Gavelin P, Hirsch JM, et al. A retrospective study of patients with mandibular fractures treated at a Swedish University Hospital 1999-2008. Ann Maxillofac Surg 2014;4(2):178–81.
9. Elhammali N, Bremerich A, Rustemeyer J. Demographical and clinical aspects of sports-related maxillofacial and skull base fractures in hospitalized patients. Int J Oral Maxillofac Surg 2010;39(9):857–62.
10. Bochlogyros PN. A retrospective study of 1,521 mandibular fractures. J Oral Maxillofac Surg 1985;13(8):597 9.
11. Chuong R, Donoff RB, Guralnick WC. A retrospective analysis of 327 mandibular fractures. J Oral Maxillofac Surg 1983;41(5):305–9.
12. Moulton-Barrett R, Rubinstein AJ, Salzhauer MA, et al. Complications of mandibular fractures. Ann Plast Surg 1998;41(3):258–63.
13. Baba J, Ohno T, Yoshida T, et al. A case of greater auricular nerve autologous nerve grafting for inferior alveolar nerve injury by mandibular fracture. Ou Daigaku Shigakushi 1989;16(1):24–30 [in Japanese].
14. Bhutia O, Kumar L, Jose A, et al. Evaluation of facial nerve following open reduction and internal fixation of subcondylar fracture through retromandibular transparotid approach. Br J Oral Maxillofac Surg 2014;52(3):236–40.
15. al-Qurainy IA, Dutton GN, Ilankovan V, et al. Midfacial fractures and the eye: the development of a system for detecting patients at risk of eye injury–a prospective evaluation. Br J Oral Maxillofac Surg 1991;29(6):368–9.
16. al-Qurainy IA, Stassen LF, Dutton GN, et al. Diplopia following midfacial fractures. Br J Oral Maxillofac Surg 1991;29(5):302–7.

17. al-Qurainy IA, Stassen LF, Dutton GN, et al. The characteristics of midfacial fractures and the association with ocular injury: a prospective study. Br J Oral Maxillofac Surg 1991;29(5):291–301.

18. Bartoli D, Fadda MT, Battisti A, et al. Retrospective analysis of 301 patients with orbital floor fracture. J Craniomaxillofac Surg 2015;43(2):244–7.

Dental and Orofacial Injuries

Paul Piccininni, BSc, DDS[a,b,c,]*, Anthony Clough, BDS (Hons LON)[a,d], Ray Padilla, DDS[e], Gabriella Piccininni, BS[f]

KEYWORDS

- Dental and orofacial injuries • Treatment • Prevention • Mouth guards

KEY POINTS

- Oral and facial injuries are very common in sport.
- Many of these injuries are preventable with proper protection.
- Proper sideline management and treatment of orofacial injuries is crucial to successful outcomes.
- Athletes have a unique set of challenges related to both oral health and dental injuries.

MODULE 1: INTRODUCTION AND INJURY STATISTICS

An unfortunate reality of participation in sport is injury. Dental and orofacial injuries are of particular concern because, unlike lacerations or fractures, they will not heal and often require an artificial or prosthetic replacement (filling, crown, implant, or denture) on a permanent basis. Also, dental injuries are expensive. The lifetime cost of an avulsed tooth in a teenage athlete can easily reach $20,000, which often exceeds the benefits available from any insurance coverage.

There are several common statistics regarding dental injuries that cross most sports. These statistics include the following:

- Approximately twice as many injuries happen in men than in women.
- Most dental injuries involve a single tooth.
- Eighty percent of all dental injuries occur in the 4 maxillary incisor teeth.
- Slightly more injuries happen to the teeth on the left side.
- There is a high incidence of repeat injuries.[1]

[a] Medical Commission – Games Group, International Olympic Committee, Lausanne, Switzerland; [b] Medical Committee, International Ice Hockey Federation, Zurich, Switzerland; [c] Mississauga Steelheads, Canadian Hockey League, Mississauga, Ontario, Canada; [d] Eastman Dental Institute, University College London, London, UK; [e] School of Dentistry, University of California, Los Angeles, Los Angeles, CA; [f] Science, Technology and Society, Stanford University, Stanford, CA
* Corresponding author. College Park, 777 Bay Street Box 111, Toronto, Ontario M5G2C8, Canada.
E-mail address: peachtor@aol.com

Clin Sports Med 36 (2017) 369–405
http://dx.doi.org/10.1016/j.csm.2016.12.001
0278-5919/17/© 2016 Elsevier Inc. All rights reserved.

Dental and orofacial injuries are very common in sport. Various studies have shown significant dental and orofacial injury rates in various sports.[2,3] However, many injury-reporting systems (IRS) do not reflect these high injury rates because of their definition of injury. If the IRS requires "the loss of a game or practice" to be reported as an injury, then a high percentage of dental injuries will not be reported because the athlete was able to return to play.

Aside from injuries, there are also concerns with the overall oral health of athletes because of issues such as travel, finances, acidic or erosive sport beverages, dehydration, and high-carbohydrate foods and snacks. During a screening of 35 athletes attending a 1998 USA Men's World Cup camp, the following results were reported:

- Thirty-three (94%) reported a previous orofacial soft tissue injury.
- Twenty (57%) reported a dental hard tissue injury.
- Six (17%) reported an avulsed tooth.
- Twenty-five (75%) were advised to seek future dental treatment.
- Six (17%) were advised to seek immediate treatment of active infection or disease.

There is no greater disappointment for an athlete than to train for years for a major competition and then be unable to participate because of a fully avoidable incident, such as a tooth infection or impacted wisdom tooth. This article is designed to help the sport physician identify, manage, and, most importantly, prevent dental and orofacial injuries and avoid any unexpected dental emergencies.

MODULE 2: ORAL HEALTH SCREENING IN THE PERIODIC HEALTH EVALUATION

Just as we ensure that cardiac and musculoskeletal examinations take place on a regular basis, it is important to consider the importance of oral health in the general well-being of an athlete. Although dental disease is rarely career or life threatening, it can and does result in many days/weeks per year of lost training and in many cases exclusion from competition.

The International Olympic Committee (IOC), in its March 2009 consensus statement, recognized the importance of a comprehensive dental examination as part of a periodic health evaluation (PHE).[4] Many national governing bodies now demand that athletes have a dental examination well before departing for the Olympic games. The IOC also provides a comprehensive dental screening program at all Summer and Winter Olympic Games in recognition of the poor oral health and high need of athletes. It is no exaggeration to say that medals have been lost in many major sports, including basketball, athletics, ice hockey, and rowing, by high-level athletes because of dental problems.

Importance of Oral Health

1. It is important to keep the athlete free from pain and pathology that could impact the ability to train and performance.
2. The athlete has the ability to train and compete at an optimal level without being compromised by dental disease or an otherwise preventable emergency.
3. Good function is essential to ensure the ability to eat, communicate, and breathe easily and correctly.
4. It maintains good aesthetics.

The role of a dental PHE is to ensure the identification and prevention of dental disease or injury.

Identify a Predisposition to Trauma

Overjet and orthodontics

An athlete with a significant overjet of the maxillary incisor teeth (in excess of 6 mm) is 3 times more likely to sustain a dental injury (**Fig. 1**). Orthodontic appliances (braces) may increase the potential risk for soft tissue injury (**Fig. 2**). **Fig. 2** also demonstrates the presence of a fixed brace in the mandibular arch, which has contributed to an alveolar plate fracture involving the 4 lower incisors, which were joined together by an arch wire. The red line adjacent to the lower right lateral incisor shows a tear in the mucosa overlying the fracture site. This image serves as a great reminder that braces do not help prevent dental injuries, as some think.

Sex

Different studies have shown that males are between 1.8 and 2.7 times more likely to sustain a dental injury in sport than females.[5]

Impacted wisdom teeth

Wisdom teeth (third molars) provide 2 potential problems for athletes. Primarily, they can become infected and swollen, severely influencing the ability to train or compete.

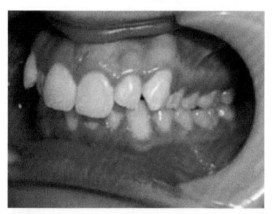

Fig. 1. Excessive overjet.

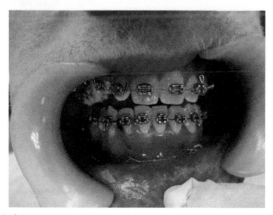

Fig. 2. Orthodontic braces.

Also, there is a much higher risk of jaw fracture if the molar is lying across the angle of the mandible between the ascending ramus and the body of the mandible (**Fig. 3**).

Wisdom teeth should be assessed between 16 and 21 years of age and, if indicated, extracted where appropriate at a time that will be least impactful on the athlete's training or competition.

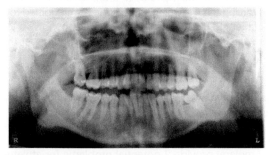

Fig. 3. Jaw fracture through wisdom tooth area.

Diagnose Oral Pathology, Including Cancer

Regular screening in athletes and the early identification of disease can minimize or prevent more serious consequences. Early detection may enable any required surgery to be scheduled around training and competition schedules.

Fig. 4 illustrates cystic changes in the mandible of an athlete identified from a routine screening examination during the Sochi Winter Olympic Games in 2014.

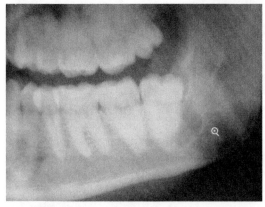

Fig. 4. Cyst around impacted wisdom tooth.

Identify Habits That May Predispose to Cancerous Change in the Oral Mucosa

Practices such as the use of chewing tobacco and betel nut as well as high-altitude outdoor training are thought to increase the risk of intraoral pathology (**Fig. 5**) as well as various lesions in the lip (**Fig. 6**).

Note the erythematous appearance, hyperkeratotic surface of the mucosa, and degree of tooth wear present in these cases. Broken teeth with sharp edges that give rise to chronic irritation may also contribute to these changes.

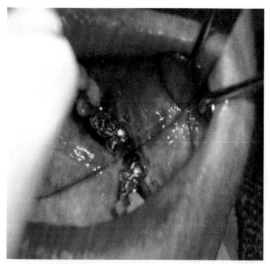

Fig. 5. Hyperkeratosis of the cheek.

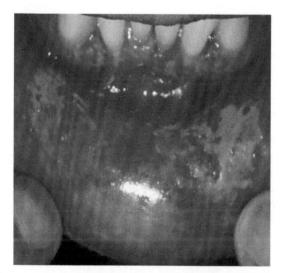

Fig. 6. Lip lesion.

Tooth Decay (Caries)

Undetected and untreated dental caries can give rise to the following:

1. Broken teeth
2. Dental infection in the surrounding tissues
3. Dental abscess in the alveolar bone
4. Ensuing postinfection bone loss
5. Tooth loss and the consequent breakdown of the occlusion
6. Pain
7. Poor appearance

Sometimes many of the aforementioned characteristics are present in the same individual (**Fig. 7**).

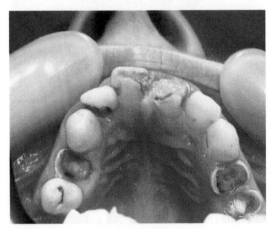

Fig. 7. Severe caries and extensive tooth destruction.

The main causes of caries in elite athletes are as follows:

1. Sport beverages
2. High sugar/carbohydrate intake
3. Poor oral hygiene
4. Lack of dental advice
5. Limited access to regular care
6. Dehydration and reduction of the protective benefits of saliva.

Periodontal (Gum) Disease

This disease may present in an acute form, such as acute ulcerative gingivitis (AUG) in (**Fig. 8**), or in the more commonly seen chronic periodontal disease (**Fig. 9**), both of which may be equally disruptive to an elite athlete.

AUG is more commonly seen in younger athletes and is caused by a bacterial infection after poor oral hygiene. *Borrelia vincentii* is commonly identified as the causative pathogen, hence, the alternative name Vincent disease.

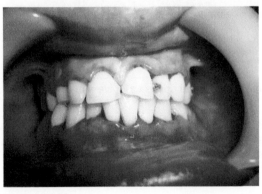

Fig. 8. Acute ulcerative gingivitis.

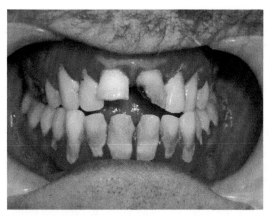

Fig. 9. Chronic periodontal disease.

AUG may be identified by the following:

1. Bleeding around the necks of the teeth
2. Necrosis of the dental papillae
3. Loss of gum contour
4. A highly offensive odor
5. General malaise

Chronic periodontal disease is widely prevalent in the older cohort of athletes and is commonly characterized by the following:

1. Severe inflammation, red angry appearance of the gingival tissues
2. Large deposits of calcified material (calculus) around the necks of the teeth
3. Bone loss causing teeth to become loose
4. Generalized inflammation of all surrounding soft tissues
5. Tooth loss with ensuing occlusal instability
6. Drifting and random movement of teeth, commonly in the incisor region
7. Bad breath

Other considerations in the periodic health evaluation

- Recognize and record any history of orofacial trauma that may be more susceptible to future damage.
- Document any previous orofacial surgery to allow appropriate protection if indicated.
- Make appropriate recommendations about mouth guards if indicated.

The goal of the dental PHE is to recognize and record any oral pathology or other conditions that might predispose the athlete to trauma or time loss due to disease or infection. It is also important to ensure that the athlete is strongly encouraged to arrange appropriate treatment of any conditions identified before participating in organized sport.

MODULE 3: SPORT BEVERAGES AND DENTAL EROSION

There has been significant recent discussion regarding the harmful effects of sport beverages on teeth, so a brief discussion of this matter and the steps that can be taken to minimize this damage is included.

Erosion of the enamel can lead to many negative results, including pulp exposure, infection, abscess, broken or lost teeth, and reduced function. The main causes of erosion include acid reflux (including that associated with eating disorders), high intake of citrus fruits or drinks, and sport beverages.

Sport-beverage consumption is increasing in athletes at all levels and is in fact encouraged by coaches and nutritionists despite the fact that these drinks have been clearly shown to be erosive in vivo.[6]

In addition to reducing the overall use of these drinks, some of the steps that athletes may consider to minimize the harmful effects include the following:

1. Dilute the drinks with bottled water.
2. Rinse the mouth with water immediately after use.
3. Use the sport beverages chilled to reduce the erosive effect.
4. Use a fluoride mouth rinse twice daily to encourage remineralization of the enamel.
5. Use special toothpastes, such as Regenerate, to promote remineralization.
6. Avoid use immediately before sleep when the buffering action of saliva will be reduced.

Dental erosion is a significant clinical problem that can be prevented and controlled by working closely with the athlete and taking appropriate proven steps.

MODULE 4: TOOTH FRACTURES

Tooth fractures are a very common and potentially devastating injury for athletes. It is imperative that the clinician be able to rapidly identify the degree of severity of the fracture, as this may determine the return-to-play status of the athlete.

The diagram in **Fig. 10** shows the basic anatomy of the tooth and supporting structures. In general terms, a fracture that involves only the enamel is usually less severe than one that enters the dentin or exposes the pulp.

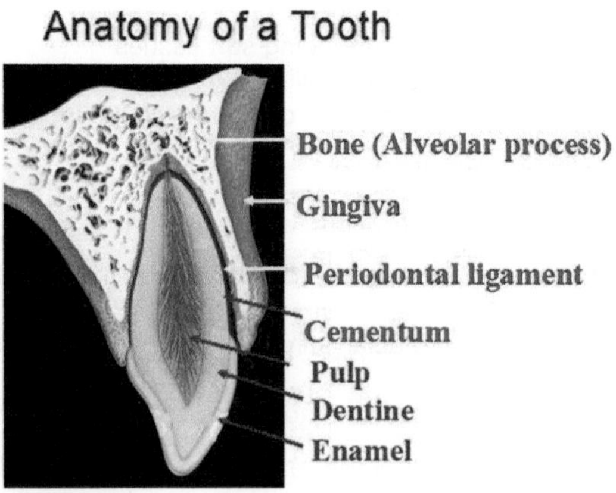

Anatomy of a Tooth

Fig. 10. Basic dental anatomy.

Please refer to the following 5 cases to gain an understanding of both the types and management of various dental fractures.

Case 1: Fracture of Enamel Only

In most cases, athletes with this type of injury can return to play. Treatment will involve restoration or reattachment of the fractured segments if retained (**Fig. 11**).

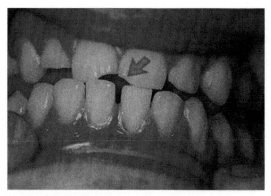

Fig. 11. Fracture of enamel only (*arrow*).

Case 2: Fracture of Enamel and Dentin, No Pulp Exposure

It is important that the missing piece be accounted for to ensure that it has not been aspirated or imbedded in the soft tissue (**Fig. 12**). If the athlete can tolerate any

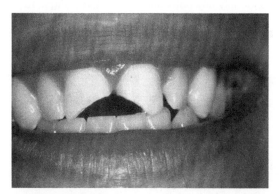

Fig. 12. Fracture of enamel and dentin.

discomfort from the exposed dentin, and the sharp edges do not put the player at any risk of soft tissue injury, then in most cases the athlete can return to play with this injury. Treatment will involve either restoration with composite resin or possible reattachment of the fractured segment.

Case 3: Fracture with Enamel Blush

A pulp (nerve) blush occurs when the underlying nerve is just slightly visible on examination (**Fig. 13**). The nerve may be marginally exposed or there may still be a very thin layer of opaque tooth structure covering the nerve. If a sideline dentist is present, this blush can be covered with a protective temporary filling and return to play may be considered. Otherwise, the athlete should be removed from competition and referred for immediate treatment to help preserve the health of the nerve and prevent infection or necrosis.

Case 4: Fracture with Pulp Exposure

When the nerve is clearly exposed, both pain and the risk of infection demand that the athlete be removed from play and referred for immediate treatment. In

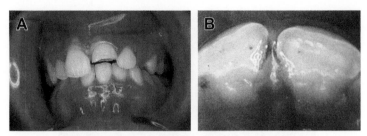

Fig. 13. (*A, B*) Tooth fractures with enamel blush.

many cases, this treatment may involve removal of the nerve, although in some cases the nerve may receive a medicated dressing and might remain vital (**Fig. 14**).

Case 5: Root Fracture

Not all tooth fractures are visible on clinical examination. Any tooth that has been traumatized, regardless of the clinical appearance, should be referred for radiographic assessment to help identify any potential root fractures (**Figs. 15–17**). The treatment and prognosis for these root-fractured teeth depends on the location of the root fracture, with fractures in the coronal third of the tooth having the worst potential for recovery.

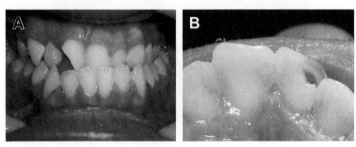

Fig. 14. (*A, B*) Fractures with pulp exposures.

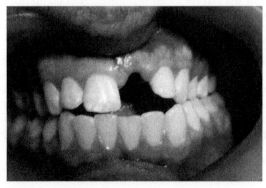

Fig. 15. Patient with severe tooth fracture.

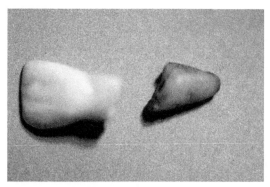

Fig. 16. Extracted tooth segments after fracture.

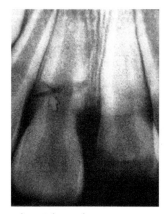

Fig. 17. Radiograph of fractured root (*arrow*).

It is crucial that the sideline physician or dentist take the time to locate all fractured tooth segments. Although often still on the field of play, these may also be imbedded in an opponents head or elbow, buried in the player's lip (**Fig. 18**), swallowed, or aspirated. Soft tissue radiographs (**Fig. 19**) may assist with identifying the location of

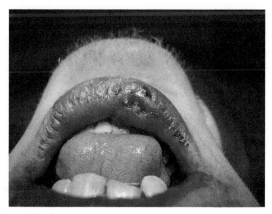

Fig. 18. Tooth fragment in lip.

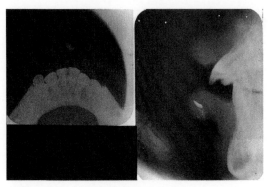

Fig. 19. Soft tissue radiograph of tooth fragment in lip.

these lost pieces. Segments that have been retrieved should be retained in a moist, semisterile solution (saline, contact lens solution, Save-a-Tooth kit) for possible reattachment.

Tooth fractures are very common in sport, and to ensure the safety of the athlete a sideline physician must be able to quickly and accurately determine the severity of the fracture and what immediate and follow-up treatment is required.[7]

MODULE 5: TOOTH LUXATION AND INTRUSION

In this section, the authors review the identification and management of a wide category of injuries to teeth that can occur after a blow, with or without fracture. These types of injuries include

- Concussion (of a tooth)
- Subluxation
- Extrusive luxation
- Lateral luxation
- Intrusive luxation (Intrusion)

Luxation injuries most commonly involve one or more of the maxillary incisors. The following discussion reviews the key feature of each type of injury.

Concussion

Concussion of the tooth results from a blow to the tooth. The tooth exhibits pain to touch, but there is no visible loosening or displacement. As with all dental injuries, it is important to view a radiographic image of the tooth, which in this case will show the tooth sitting normally in the socket. The radiograph will help confirm the lack of a root fracture.

In most cases it is appropriate for athletes to return to play without any greater risk of further damage occurring. Pulp necrosis and loss of vitality is a rare but occasional occurrence with these injuries.

Subluxation

This term describes an injury to one or more of the maxillary incisors that results in limited mobility without any visible displacement. It is not uncommon to see hemorrhage in the gingival sulcus around the neck of the crown of the tooth (**Fig. 20**).

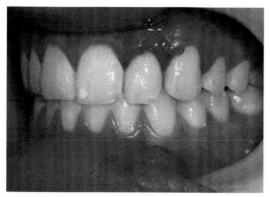

Fig. 20. Subluxation with bleeding around tooth.

Return to play in these cases is a matter of judgment, depending primarily on the degree of mobility of the tooth and whether in the opinion of the physician the tooth is at an increased risk of falling out. In sports where mouth guards are routinely worn, there would be little danger in returning to play wearing a guard. However, for players not wearing a mouth guard and who are playing in high-contact positions or sports, the injury risk may preclude a return to play until the tooth has been stabilized and protected.

Treatment may involve a minor alteration to the player's occlusion by the team dentist. Additionally the player might be advised to adopt a softer diet for 2 to 3 weeks while healing of the tissues supporting the teeth occurs. In some cases it may be necessary for the dentist to splint the teeth for up to 3 weeks (**Fig. 21**). A mouth guard should be worn if return to play is considered in these more severe cases. It can easily be fitted around any splint.

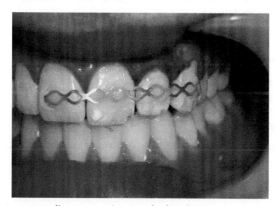

Fig. 21. Titanium trauma splint supporting tooth. (Medartis AG, Basel, Switzerland.)

Where hemorrhage is observed around the neck of the teeth, a course of antibiotics is advised to reduce the likelihood of ingress of bacteria down the root and into the periodontal ligament (**Fig. 22**). Antibacterial oral rinses are also indicated.

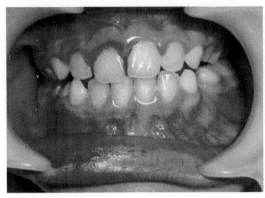

Fig. 22. Bleeding around sulcus of tooth.

Prognosis

In most cases healing occurs without any further complications. However, the stage of root development and the presence of any crown fracture may determine the potential for pulp death (**Fig. 23**).

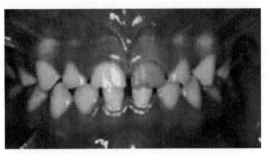

Fig. 23. Discolored tooth following trauma.

With all luxation injuries the following may occur:

1. Darkened tooth as a result of pulp death
2. Dental abscess following damage of the pulp tissues
3. Loss of bone in the surrounding areas
4. Root resorption

Appropriate follow-up appointments following the initial injury will help identify these sequelae at an early stage and limit the resulting damage.

Extrusive Luxation

Extrusive luxation (as the name suggests) describes a situation whereby one or more teeth are partially displaced (extruded) out of the tooth socket (**Fig. 24**).[8]

When an extrusive injury has occurred, the teeth appear longer and are often tilted toward the palate (**Fig. 25**). In all cases they will be significantly loosened as the periodontal ligament has been torn or ruptured and the neurovascular bundle at the tip has been severed. At this stage the tooth is often relying only on the surrounding tissue to hold it in place.

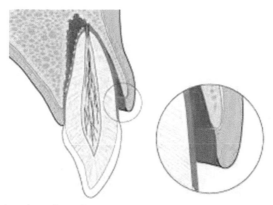

Fig. 24. Extrusive luxation of tooth.

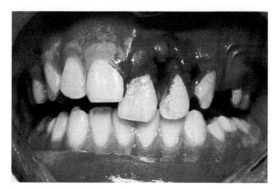

Fig. 25. Extrusive luxation of multiple teeth.

Treatment

The teeth should be gently pushed back up into their sockets. It is not normally necessary to administer a local anesthetic, and this procedure may be undertaken at the side of the field of play. During the process of pushing the tooth into the socket, the blood clot may be extruded (**Fig. 26**) out from the area around the neck of the tooth (gingival crevice) and should not cause any concern.

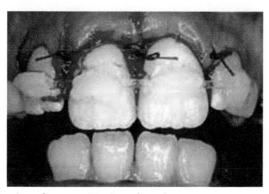

Fig. 26. Blood extrusion after repositioning of tooth.

The tooth/teeth may have also been pushed palatally and may need to be pulled forward with your fingertips at the same time that they are being pushed back into their sockets. If the teeth are to be saved, it is important that the athlete does not return to play but instead goes immediately to a dentist to have the teeth splinted into the correct position.

Antibiotics should be given as a precaution to prevent the invasion of bacteria down the periodontal ligament.

Prognosis

In children, where the tooth apex is open, the pulp will often revascularize and the tooth remains vital. **Figs. 27–30** show repositioning and splinting of a tooth with an open apex in a child. In adults, however, pulp death most commonly occurs.

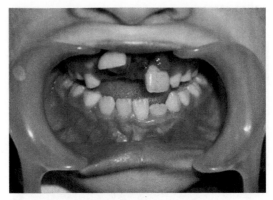

Fig. 27. Severe tooth luxation in a young patient.

Complications

The complications that could occur include the following:

1. Pulp death (dark tooth)
2. Loss of the surrounding bone
3. Root resorption
4. Possible infection
5. Lost tooth if not held in place

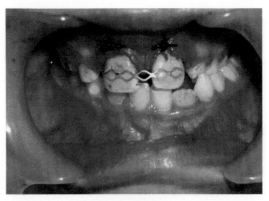

Fig. 28. Following reposition, suturing and splinting.

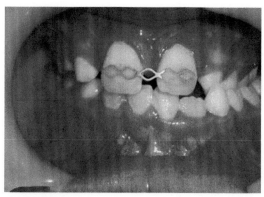

Fig. 29. After soft tissue healing.

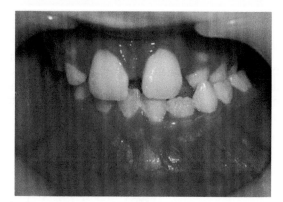

Fig. 30. Final result after splint removal.

Lateral Luxation

Although called a lateral luxation, this injury may be either a lateral or anterior/posterior displacement of one or more teeth and is often accompanied by a fracture of the alveolar plate. In cases whereby several teeth are involved, they may all move as one unit where they are attached to the alveolar bone plate. In **Figs. 31** and **32**, the 4 mandibular incisors have been pushed backward (lingual) as a single unit (see **Fig. 12**).

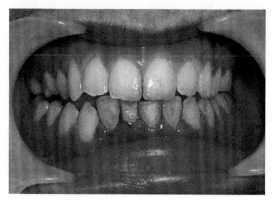

Fig. 31. Lateral luxation of 4 incisors.

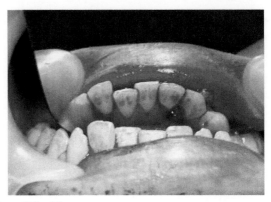

Fig. 32. Mirror view of **Fig. 31**.

Unlike other luxation injuries, the tooth remains solid in its socket as it is firmly attached to the bone. Classically, the root apex of the tooth moves anteriorly (**Figs. 33** and **34**) as the crown of the tooth is struck and is moved palatally. The root apex fractures through the anterior alveolar wall and remains locked or wedged between the socket and the newly fractured alveolar plate.

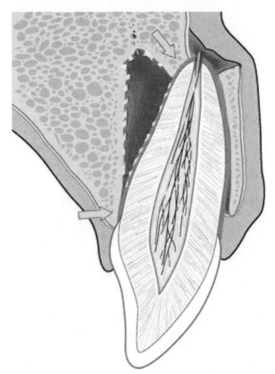

Fig. 33. Apex of tooth with anterior movement (*arrows* indicate extensive movement at apex vs collar of tooth).

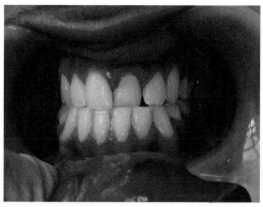

Fig. 34. Clinical case of lateral luxation.

It may sometimes be possible to palpate the root apex and even the fractured bony plate by running a finger along the labial sulcus.

Treatment

The displaced tooth is normally firmly wedged into its new position and requires substantial force to reposition it from where it has become lodged.

Local anesthetic is normally necessary for this painful procedure, which involves applying force in an incisal tip direction using fingers or in some cases forceps. There is often a noticeable click as the tooth disengages followed by a second click as it lodges back into its socket.

The tooth requires splinting by the team dentist for a minimum of 4 weeks, which will allow the alveolar fracture to heal. If a group of teeth have been luxated, care must be taken if marginal breakdown has occurred at the bone margins. If this occurs, 6 to 8 weeks of splinting may be necessary. Appropriate antibiotics should be given to prevent bacterial infection at the fracture site.

Prognosis

Revascularization of the pulp is unlikely, and pulp death can be expected. Root treatment of the affected teeth should be considered at the same time as splinting. Root resorption may occur, but it is a rare occurrence. Follow-up for at least 1 year after injury is suggested.

Intrusive Luxation/Intrusion

This luxation/intrusion involves the displacement of the tooth apically through the floor of the tooth socket. It is normally associated with a comminution or fracture of the alveolar socket (**Fig. 35**). The position of the tooth should be confirmed radiographically.

Intrusive injuries comprise approximately 2% of all dental trauma and often have the most severe consequences. Intruded teeth are extremely firm where they have been forced into the socket and will always result in pulp death, and often root surface resorption, because of the severity of the damage to the neurovascular bundle and periodontal ligament.

Oral bacteria forced into the socket by the force of the injury present a real risk of infection in the damaged area, and antibiotics should be given routinely. In general an intrusive injury has the worst prognosis of all the luxations (see **Fig. 13B**).

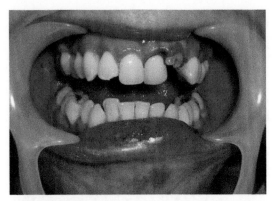

Fig. 35. Intrusion of lateral incisor.

Treatment

As the tooth is firmly positioned in the socket, it may be possible for the athlete to return to the field of play. Spontaneous resorption of intruded teeth is unreliable, and the tooth should be repositioned either orthodontically (**Fig. 36**) or surgically as soon as possible. Repositioning should be followed by splinting (**Fig. 37**).

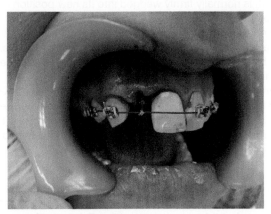

Fig. 36. Orthodontic extrusion of intruded tooth.

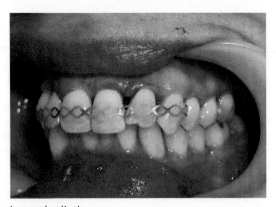

Fig. 37. Repositioning and splinting.

Complications

If left untreated the tooth may

1. Darken
2. Become ankylosed (fused) with the bone and impossible to move
3. Become infected

A fully intruded tooth may result in the root tip being forced into the nasal cavity. Clinical and radiographic examination of the nasal cavity can confirm if this has occurred. Surgical repositioning of the tooth is the treatment of choice is these cases.

MODULE 6: DENTAL AVULSIONS

Dental avulsion is the complete traumatic displacement of a tooth from the alveolar (bony) socket (**Figs. 38** and **39**). Treatment is immediate replacement and stabilization of the avulsed tooth back into the socket. Primary (deciduous teeth) should not be replanted because of the risk of damage to the adult tooth bud.

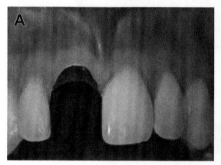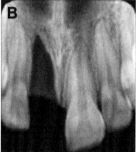

Fig. 38. (*A, B*) Avulsions of teeth from socket.

In sports, this injury is best prevented by the use of helmets, face shields, and properly fitted professionally made mouth guards when applicable. It is essential that the athletic mouth guards fit properly and are not displaced on impact. This requirement would rule out the over-the-counter, store-bought variety of mouth guards.

The immediate treatment (ideally within 5 minutes) of the avulsion dictates the success of the treatment. Therefore, it is necessary for the caregiver, coach, parent, or school nurse to begin replantation treatment before the arrival at an emergency facility or dental office.

The avulsed tooth should be handled by the crown of the tooth (**Fig. 40**) and not the root. It should be quickly rinsed (not scrubbed) with cold water, saline, or milk and immediately placed back into the bony socket. If the avulsed tooth is not immediately placed back into the socket, coagulation or blood clotting of the avulsed bony socket may prevent the tooth from being replaced into its original position.

Kenny and colleagues[9] strongly recommended that replantation be done within the first 5 minutes following the injury for best results. Do not wait for the dentist or emergency personnel. Replant at the site of the injury. The drying of the cells on the root surface drastically reduces success. If you cannot replant immediately, place the tooth in physiologic saline, milk, or Hanks Balanced Salt Solution. Milk is often the most readily available solution. Do not store in water. Water has been shown to damage the tooth root periodontal ligament cells. The osmolality and pH of water is very low compared with normal cell pressure and will cause the periodontal ligament cells of the root to become damaged.

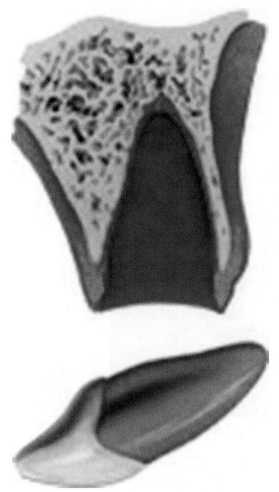

Fig. 39. Image of tooth avulsion. (*Courtesy of* the Dental Trauma Guide, dental traumaguide.org.)

If the injured person is unconscious, do not attempt to replant the tooth for fear of aspiration. Await total consciousness before replanting by storing the tooth as recommended earlier. Once the tooth has been replanted, immediately take the injured athlete to a qualified trauma dentist for splinting of the teeth and suturing of gingival lacerations (if necessary).

On arrival at the dental office, the dentist will radiograph the avulsed area, apply a flexible splint, and initiate and complete root canal treatment. The treatment material of choice for splinting is a titanium trauma splint with composite flowable resin. The splint is kept in for 2 weeks or longer depending on the severity of the injury and damage to the alveolar bone (**Fig. 41**).

If needed, systemic antibiotics (clindamycin or amoxicillin) may be prescribed as well as checking for tetanus prophylaxis status. After an appropriate time, the splint can be removed. Continue to monitor the tooth at 6 months and yearly.[9]

External inflammatory resorption and replacement resorption are factors that may present themselves years after the avulsion injury. This negative result is more likely to occur the longer the avulsed tooth was kept out of the mouth and is also related to

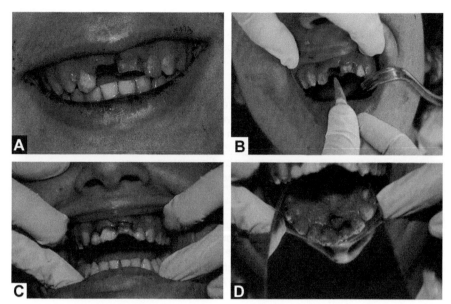

Fig. 40. (*A*) Avulsed central incisor tooth. (*B*) Replanting tooth holding crown only. (*C–D*) Replantation and soft tissue closure. (*From* Tezel H, Atalayin C, Kayrak G. Replantation after traumatic avulsion. Eur J Dent 2013;7:229–32; with permission.)

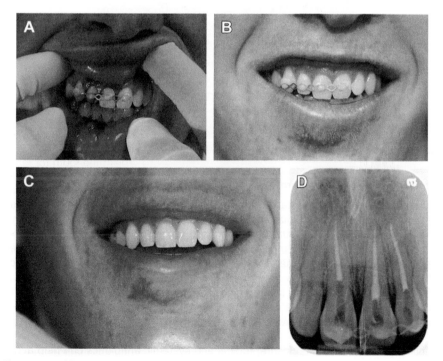

Fig. 41. Avulsion case sequencing (*A*) Immediate splinting; (*B*) 2 weeks Postoperative; (*C*) splint removal; (*D*) postoperative radiographs. (*Courtesy* of Dr Ray Padilla, DDS.)

the storage medium used before replantation. This replacement resorption may ultimately result in the loss of the tooth. That is why it is critical to replant the tooth immediately at the site of injury and complete root canal therapy within a few days of the injury.

MODULE 7: SOFT TISSUE INJURIES

Intraoral, perioral, and facial lacerations are all common occurrences in competitive and recreational sport. Athletes who have uncontrolled bleeding are usually not allowed to return to play for both their own safety and the safety of their opponent.

As with other lacerations, proper debridement and, where indicated, a layered closure will help to ensure proper healing and a quick recovery.

Please refer to the following 4 cases to review the management of various soft tissue injuries.

Uncomplicated External Laceration

This laceration includes a foreign body (tooth segment) that must be removed and retained for possible reattachment. Removal of any small salivary glands is good practice (**Fig. 42**). The use of tissue adhesives, after closure with sutures, and ice to reduce postoperative swelling is often suggested. Antibiotics may be indicated.

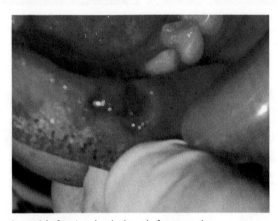

Fig. 42. Lip laceration with foreign body (tooth fragment).

Deep Laceration/Vermilion Border

This case very likely requires stabilization at the field of play and then a referral to plastics for proper closure to minimize scarring (**Fig. 43**). However, it does illustrate several key considerations in the closure of more severe oral lacerations. Any tear involving the vermilion border of the lip must be carefully closed to avoid a step in the border after healing. Closure should start by approximating the edges of the vermilion border before closing any other areas.

Also, deep lesions require a layered closure to minimize dead space and properly approximate the tissues. This deep layer should be thoroughly cleaned and then closed with resorbable sutures. Any small, unsupported saliva glands can be removed to promote healing. Once closed, external closure can begin with the vermilion border. Following closure, topical and systemic antibiotics can help avoid infection and also keep the tissues moist. Ice and antiinflammatory medications are imperative.

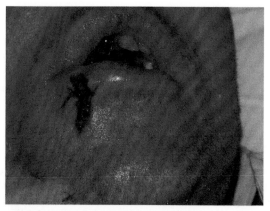

Fig. 43. Deep laceration requiring extensive layered closure.

Intraoral Laceration/Through-and-Through

In any case whereby the intraoral mucosa or tongue is lacerated, it is proper practice to close these lacerations to restore proper anatomy, reduce healing time, and prevent infection (**Fig. 44**). Many practitioners have been advised that, because one cannot sterilize the site before closure, these intraoral lacerations should be left open to reduce the risk of postoperative infection. This notion is not true. Proper closure, often in combination with an antibacterial rinse, is the proper treatment, as indicated later.

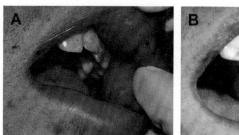 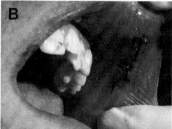

Fig. 44. (*A*, *B*) Before and after closure of intraoral laceration.

Degloving and Gingival Trauma

It is not uncommon for the gingival tissues to be stripped back causing a degloving injury (**Fig. 45**). As with other soft tissue injuries, these tissues should be properly cleaned and debrided and then closed to help retain both proper anatomy and

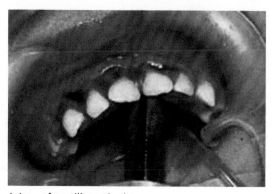

Fig. 45. Degloving injury of maxillary gingiva.

coverage of the tooth root and alveolus. Following closure, a periodontal pack might be placed and topical antibacterial rinses along with a soft diet are indicated.

Sport physicians have been trained to leave many intraoral lacerations open because the area cannot be rendered reasonably bacteria free before closure. To promote proper healing and to retain proper soft tissue architecture, most intraoral and tongue lacerations should be sutured.

MODULE 8: TEMPOROMANDIBULAR JOINT INJURIES

The most common temporomandibular joint (TMJ) injuries in sport are fractures of the condyle and subluxation of the joint. When this joint is subluxed, it is imperative that the sideline physician make a prompt effort to reposition this joint back into place before muscle spasm makes this impossible without hospitalization and sedation.

The TMJ is the only joint in the body capable of both translation and rotation, which is accomplished by means of the articular disc (**Fig. 46**). When the ligaments supporting this disc have been traumatized, the athlete may have clicking, popping, or locking of the joint. Treatment requires a proper diagnosis and radiographs or other imaging if indicated as well as therapy, medications, and diet considerations.

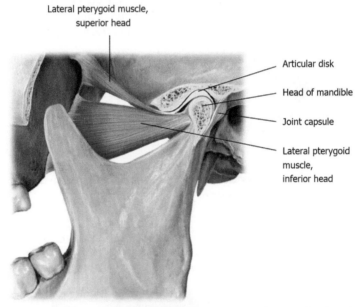

Fig. 46. Anatomy of TMJ. (*From* Gilroy AM, Macpherson BR, Ross LM, et al. Atlas of anatomy. New York: Thieme, 2012; with permission.)

Any blow to the jaw can lead to a subluxation of the joint. Once it has been determined that there is no fracture present, the joint should be repositioned as quickly as possible to help prevent trismus. A gentle downward and backward force will usually encourage the condylar head to slip over the articular eminence and return to the fossa.

Postinjury management following reposition would include ice, antiinflammatory medications, minimizing opening for 5 to 7 days, a soft diet, and appropriate physiotherapy.

TMJ injuries can become chronic and debilitating injuries if not identified and managed properly. A team approach, which includes dental assessment and splinting if indicated, nutrition counseling, and physiotherapy, provides the best solution for the injured athlete.

MODULE 9: MAXILLARY AND MANDIBULAR FRACTURES

In many high-impact and heavy-collision sports, maxillary and mandibular fractures are an unfortunate reality. These injuries can be season ending and, on occasion, life threatening; their identification and proper management is an important tool for the sideline physician.

Maxillary Fractures

The two most common maxillary fractures in sport are segmental fractures and Le Fort I.

Segmental fractures (**Fig. 47**) can be diagnosed both clinically and radiographically. In most cases, there would be instability and mobility in more than one tooth, unlike a single-tooth luxation injury. Treatment in most cases consists of rigid stabilization of the fracture for a minimum of 4 to 6 weeks. This stabilization can usually be accomplished by means of a fixed wire bonded to the adjacent teeth, although in some severe cases intraosseous fixation may be required.

A rare but serious maxillary fracture is the Le Fort I fracture (**Fig. 48**). This fracture can occur after a severe anterior blow to the maxilla from a head, elbow, or goalpost. The

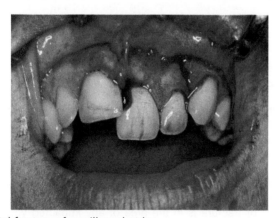

Fig. 47. Segmental fracture of maxillary alveolus.

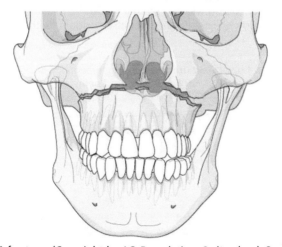

Fig. 48. Le Fort 1 fracture. (Copyright by AO Foundation, Switzerland. Source: AO Surgery Reference, www.aosurgery.org.)

greatest concern to the sideline physician is the instability of the fracture and the potential for closing the airway, as the fractured maxilla can drop posteriorly. In this situation, the sideline physician must reposition the maxilla anteriorly to open up the airway.

Mandibular Fractures

Aside from segmental fractures, which would in most cases be managed in a similar manner to maxillary fractures, the 3 most common mandibular fractures are body, ramus, and condylar fractures (**Fig. 49**).

Often, the fracture can be predicted from the nature of the facial blow. For example,

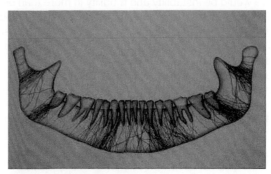

Fig. 49. Typical fracture lines in mandible.

a severe blow to the chin point is most likely to result in a fracture at either the point of contact and/or in the condyle area. A blow to the side of the face often results in a fracture at either the point of contact and/or the contralateral condyle or ramus. As these secondary fractures, away from the point of contact, can readily be missed, proper radiographic imaging is imperative.

Management of these fractures can include nonsurgical conservative treatment, extraoral fixation, or surgical stabilization.

A common point of fracture is in the area of any impacted wisdom tooth (third molar). Some studies have cited a 2 to 4 times greater incidence of mandibular fracture in athletes with impacted wisdom teeth (**Fig. 50**).[10,11] Athletes in contact sports such as football should consider having impacted wisdom teeth removed during the off-season.

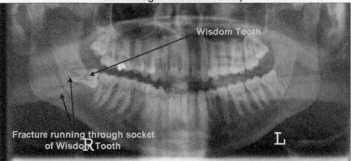

Fig. 50. Mandibular fracture associated with impacted right wisdom tooth.

Any athlete suffering a severe blow to the maxilla or mandible must be referred for appropriate imaging. Not all of these fractures have reliable clinical symptoms, and can often be missed during a clinical examination.

MODULE 10: INJURY PREVENTION AND ATHLETIC MOUTH GUARDS

Properly diagnosed, designed, and custom fabricated mouth guards are essential to the prevention of athletic oral/facial injuries.

In Flanders and Bhat's[12] 1995 study, they reported on the high incidence of injuries in sports other than football. In American football, where mouth guards are worn, 0.07% of the injuries were orofacial. In basketball where mouth guards are not routinely worn, 34% of the injuries were orofacial.[12] Various degrees of injury, from simple contusions and lacerations to avulsions and fractured jaws, were reported.

The National Youth Sports Foundation for the Prevention of Athletic Injuries reports several interesting statistics. Dental injuries are the most common type of orofacial injury sustained during participation in sports. Victims of total tooth avulsions who do not have teeth properly preserved or replanted may face lifetime dental costs of up to $20,000 per tooth, hours in the dentist's chair, and the possible development of other dental problems, such as periodontal disease.

It is estimated by the American Dental Association that mouth guards prevent approximately 200,000 injuries each year in high school and collegiate football alone.

A properly fitted mouth guard must be protective, comfortable, resilient, tear resistant, odorless, tasteless, not bulky, cause minimal interference to speaking and breathing, and (possibly the most important criteria) have excellent retention, fit, and sufficient thickness in critical areas.

Unfortunately, the word *mouth guard* is universal and generic and includes a large range and variety of products, from over-the-counter models bought at the sporting goods stores to professionally manufactured and dentist-prescribed custom-made mouth guards.

Presently, more than 90% of the mouth guards worn are of the variety bought at sporting good stores. The other 10% are of the custom-made variety diagnosed and designed by a health professional (dentist and/or athletic trainer).

There are 4 types of mouth guards presently available. Each type is discussed.

Stock mouth guard: The stock mouth guard (**Fig. 51**), available at most sporting good stores, comes in limited sizes (usually small, medium, and large) and is the least expensive and least protective. The price ranges from $3 to $30. These protectors are

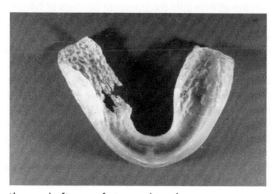

Fig. 51. Stock mouth guard after use for several weeks.

ready to be used without any further preparation; simply remove from the package and immediately place in the mouth. They are bulky and lack any retention and, therefore, must be held in place by constantly biting down. This mouth guard interferes with speech and breathing, making the stock mouth guard the least acceptable and least protective. This type of mouth guard is often altered and cut by the athlete in an attempt to make it more comfortable, further reducing the protective properties of the mouth guard. It has been suggested and advised in the medical/dental literature that these types of mouth guards not be worn because of their lack of retention and protective properties.

As sports dentists and health professionals interested in injury prevention, the authors do not recommend this type of mouth guard to their patients and athletic teams.

Mouth-formed or boil-and-bite mouth guard: Presently, this is the most commonly used mouth guard on the market. Most marketing and advertising in the past has been for this type of mouth guard. Made from thermoplastic material, they are immersed in boiling water and formed in the mouth by using finger, tongue, and biting pressure. Available in limited sizes, these mouth guards often lack proper extensions and often do not cover all the posterior teeth. Dental mouth-arch-length studies have shown that most boil-and-bite mouth guards do not cover all posterior teeth in most high school and collegiate athletes (**Fig. 52**). Athletes also cut and alter these bulky and ill-fitting

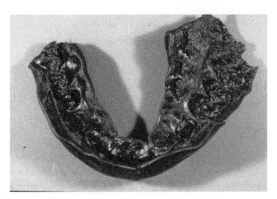

Fig. 52. Boil-and-bite mouth guard after usage.

boil-and-bite mouth guards because of their poor fit, poor retention, and gagging effects. This practice, in turn, further reduces the minimal protective properties of these mouth guards. When the athlete cuts the posterior borders or bites through the mouth guard during forming, they increase their chance of injury. Certain thicknesses and extensions are necessary for proper mouth guard protection.

Dr Hunter,[13] a noted Australian sports dentist, reported that mouth guards should be of certain thickness, without being bulky. He suggests labial thickness of 3 mm, palatal thickness of 2 mm, and occlusal thickness of 3 mm. The mouth guard material should be biocompatible and have good physical properties. These thicknesses are recommended thicknesses. It should be noted that each athlete should be evaluated individually for thickness and design as to promote comfort and sufficient protection.

Dr Park and colleagues,[14] reported that boil-and-bite mouth guards provide a false sense of protection because of the dramatic decrease in thickness occlusally during the molding and fabrication process. They reported that boil-and-bite mouth guards decrease in occlusal thickness 70% to 99% during molding, thus taking away most of the protective properties of the mouth guard.

Care should be taken by the public when bombarded with clever marketing schemes, claims, and promotions by stock and boil-and-bite mouth guard companies. The bottom line is that stock and boil-and-bite mouth guards do not provide the expected care and injury prevention that a properly diagnosed and fabricated custom-made mouth guard does. Why is there a general belief that mouth guards are uncomfortable, do not fit, are bulky, and interfere with breathing and speaking? Could it be because 90% of today's mouth guards worn are of the stock or boil-and-bite variety and it is the perception by the public and coaches that these are the only available mouth guards? Indeed, most mouth guards today do not fit, are bulky, and do interfere with speaking and breathing because they are wearing stock or boil-and-bite mouth guards from the sporting goods stores. Most athletes are not wearing properly made dentally diagnosed and designed custom-made mouth guards provided by a sports dentist.

Sports dentists and health professionals interested in injury prevention do not recommend store bought boil-and-bite mouth guards to their patients and athletic teams. The public deserves the best quality of care in injury prevention, and boil-and-bite mouth guards DO NOT provide this quality.

Custom-made mouth guard: Custom-made mouth guards are supplied by a dentist. Custom mouth guards provide the dentist with the critical ability to address several important issues in the fitting of the mouth guard. Several questions must be answered before the custom mouth guard can be fabricated. These questions include those addressed at the preseason screening or dental examination.

1. Is the mouth guard designed for the particular sport being played?
2. Is the age of the athlete and the possibility of providing space for erupting teeth in mixed dentition (aged 6–12 years) going to affect the mouth guard?
3. Will the design of the mouth guard be appropriate for the level of competition being played?
4. Does the patient have any history of previous dental injury, thus, needing additional protection in any specific area?
5. Is the athlete undergoing orthodontic treatment?
6. Does the patient present with cavities and/or missing teeth?
7. Is the athlete being helped by a dentist and/or athletic trainer or by a sporting good retailer not trained in medical/dental issues?

These questions are important questions that the sporting goods store retailer and the boil-and-bite mouth guard CANNOT begin to address.

Custom-made mouth guards are designed by a dentist and are the most satisfactory of all types of mouth protectors. They fulfill all the criteria for adaptation, retention, comfort, and stability of material. They interfere the least with speaking, and studies have shown that the custom-made mouth guards have virtually no negative effect on breathing.

There are 2 categories of custom mouth guards, the vacuum mouth guard and the pressure-laminated mouth guard.

The *vacuum mouth guard* is made from a stone cast of the mouth, usually of the maxillary (upper) arch, using an impression (mold) fabricated by a dentist. A thermoplastic mouth guard material is adapted over the cast with a special vacuum machine.

The most common material for this use is a polyethylene vinyl acetate (EVA) copolymer. The vacuum mouth guard is then trimmed and polished to allow for proper tooth and gum adaptation. Posterior teeth should be covered and muscle attachments unimpinged. Vacuum machines are adequate for single-layer mouth guards. However, it is now being shown in the dental literature that multiple-layer mouth guards (laboratory pressure laminated) may be preferred to the single-layer vacuum mouth guards.

It should be noted that these vacuum custom mouth guards are still superior to the store bought stock and boil-and-bite mouth guards because they have a much better fit, are made from a mold of your mouth, and are designed by your dentist.

Strap attachments to helmets may be requested and are easily adapted to the custom-made mouth guard, although not needed because of the better fit. Custom-made mouth guards can be fabricated through the dental office or commercial laboratory for a nominal fee.

A *custom-made multiple-layered mouth guard* is the best mouth guard available today. This pressure-laminated mouth guard can be modified for full contact sports by laminating 2 or 3 layers of EVA material to achieve the optimal thickness. Lamination is defined as the layering of mouth guard material to achieve a defined end result and thickness under a high-heat and pressure environment. Efficient and complete lamination cannot be achieved under low heat and vacuum. The layers will not properly fuse together with the vacuum machine but will chemically fuse and properly adapt under high heat and pressure with machines, such as the Drufomat (Drufomat Inc, Unna, Germany) (**Fig. 53**), the Erkopress (Erkopress Inc, Pfalzgrafenweiler, Germany) (**Fig. 54**), or the Biostar (Biostar Inc, Iserlohn, Germany) (**Fig. 55**).

Protective thickness is important because as the thickness of the mouth guard material increases, the transmitted impact force decreases. In addition to adequate thickness, the mouth guard material should be biocompatible, have good physical properties, and last for at least 2 years. It should be noted that each athlete should be evaluated individually for thickness and design to ensure both comfort and sufficient protection.

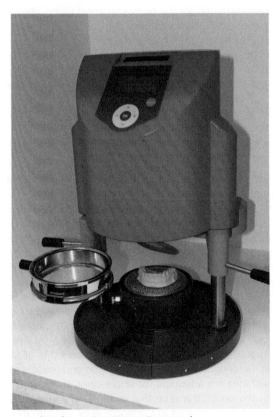

Fig. 53. Drufomat scan. (Drufomat Inc, Unna, Germany.)

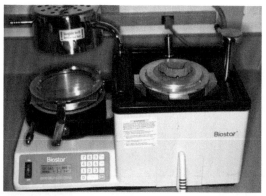

Fig. 54. Biostar. (Biostar Inc, Iserlohn, Germany.)

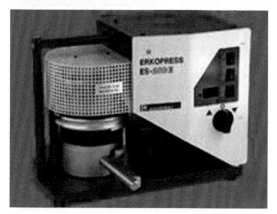

Fig. 55. Erkopress. (Erkopress Inc, Pfalzgrafenweiler, Germany.)

Pressure Thermoformed Laminated Mouth Guards

The clear advantages of pressure-formed lamination include the following:

- There is precise adaptation (**Fig. 56**).
- There is negligible deformation when worn for a period of time. The combination of the relatively high heat and pressure used in construction of laminated mouth guards means that the mouth guard material has virtually no elastic memory.

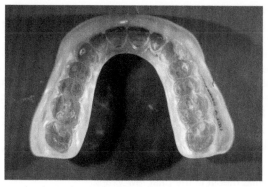

Fig. 56. Clear pressure-laminated mouth guard. (*Courtesy of* Dr Ray Padilla, DDS.)

- There is the ability to thicken any area as required as well as to place any inserts that may be needed for additional wearer protection (**Fig. 57**).

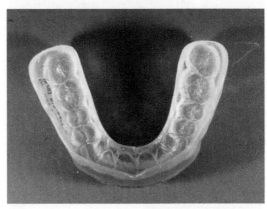

Fig. 57. Pressure-laminated guard with additional anterior layer. (*Courtesy of* Dr Ray Padilla, DDS.)

Mouth guards must maintain minimal and consistent thicknesses in critical areas. These thicknesses vary according to the athletes individual needs for optimal protection in their sport. The thicker materials (3–4 mm) are more effective in absorbing impact energy, and the thinner materials show marked deformation at the site of impact. These mouth guards are not bulky and uncomfortable.

The clinician cannot expect that a 3-mm thick material will remain 3 mm thick after fabrication. This idea is a physical impossibility because of shrinkage during fabrication adaptation. Vacuuming a commercially laminated 3-mm sheet of EVA will give the same unsatisfactory results. Therefore, laboratory pressure-lamination procedures must be used incorporating 2 or more EVA materials to achieve the end result of 3 mm to 4 mm thickness occlusally, which will allow the clinician to monitor and measure these results before delivery of these mouth guards.

There are presently 2 ways of obtaining a pressure-laminated mouth guard: dentist fabrication with the Drufomat scan, Erkopress, or Biostar in the dental office or referral to a qualified commercial laboratory presently using the pressure lamination technique.

In cases whereby dentists do not wish to construct the pressure-laminated mouth guard in their office, there are laboratories that fabricate the pressure-laminated mouth guard. Most sports dentists dealing with elite athletes recommend the custom-made mouth guard, especially those of the laboratory-lamination type for the very best in oral/facial protection.

This section presents a discussion of the various issues relating to injury prevention and mouth guards. By acknowledging these significant differences in mouth guards, the public will be better informed and educated to seek their dentistry from dental health professionals and not from sporting goods retailers.

MODULE 11: OTHER ISSUES IN SPORT DENTISTRY

This section looks into two topics that have received significant attention in both the popular and scientific media in the past few years.

Do Mouth Guards Prevent Concussion?

Many mouth guard manufacturers have made claims regarding the ability of their product to reduce either the incidence or severity of concussions. Mouth guards with names like "Brain-pad" have used the concussion epidemic in sport to sell their products. Some articles have been produced citing mainly, if not exclusively, anecdotal evidence only. What are the claims being made, and do they have any validity?

How might mouth guards play a role in reducing concussions?

There are generally 3 theories that are presented to help validate these claims. These are as follows:

1. Dissipation of force
2. Reduction of impact to the TMJ complex
3. Head stabilization using the mouth guard

Dissipation of force This argument proposes that a properly designed mouth guard, with adequate thickness and coverage of all the teeth, will have a large area of EVA material that can both absorb and dissipate the force of an upward blow to the jaw.

Reduction of impact to the temporomandibular joint complex When wearing a properly fitted mouth guard, the space between the head of the condyle and the skull is increased. At impact, this space increase may be enough to reduce or prevent any impact between the condylar head and temporal fossa.

Head stabilization When biting down hard on a mouth guard, the athlete may activate the head and neck muscles to the degree that, on impact, the rotational forces on the head may be reduced and the head may in fact go through a smaller arc of rotation. These rotational forces have been theorized as being particularly harmful in concussion severity.

Current Status of Mouth Guard/Concussion Issue

1. US Federal Trade Commission (FTC): In 2012, the US FTC fined one company and warned many others that they could no longer advertise the fact that their mouth guards prevented concussion. This action has obviously reduced, and almost eliminated, these claims over the past 2 years.
2. Academy for Sport Dentistry: See the later discussion.
3. Concussion in Sports Group: This group of highly recognized scientists and physicians have met on 5 occasions and have produced the current guidelines on categorization of concussion, return to play, and so forth. The mouth guard issue has been addressed in their statements as well as in a separate article by Co-Chairman Dr Paul McCrory.[15] Their position can be summarized as follows: There is currently no scientific evidence that confirms any relationship between concussions and mouth guard use.[16] However, McCrory[15] clearly states that "absence of proof is not proof of absence." Recent research (2016) has shed new light on a possible beneficial role of mouth guards in concussion prevention.

Do Mouth Guards Play a Role in Performance Enhancement?

Another wave of both researchers and manufacturers have spent the last few years attempting to sell their mouth guards to athletes with claims of performance enhancement.

These claims are based on several different theories, which include the following:

1. Mouth guard use allowing the jaw to reposition anteriorly, opening up the airway and improving breathing
2. Realignment of a malpositioned jaw to a more harmonious position, which may allow improved function of associated supporting structures
3. Discussions on the various levels of cortisol release with and without mouth guards, and the effect this may have on performance

One valid argument related to performance enhancement is found when a mouth guard or splint is used to stabilize a jaw that, during the associated activity, is put into an odd or unstable position. This activity may include sports like downhill skiing or cycling, whereby the body position puts the jaw in a very unharmonious position.

Another possible performance enhancement occurs with weight and power lifters. These athletes feel the need to clench down hard in order to stabilize their head and neck and maximize the power being delivered. They can do so without fear of breaking teeth by wearing a splint or guard, and many athletes do so.

However, at this time there is no clear evidence of performance improvement related to mouth guard use. In fact, the National Athletic Trainers Association, in their 2016 position statement, clearly state that:

"Properly fitted mouthguards can be used by athletes in both aerobic and anaerobic sports. Use of these devices has no negative effect on breathing or strength. Likewise, mouthguards should not be recommended to athletes to improve performance, as no high-quality evidence supports this claim."[17]

There is no science that supports the use of mouth guards in sports for either concussion prevention or performance enhancement. However, there is abundant validated scientific evidence regarding the benefit of mouth guards in preventing dental and oral injuries in sports. Mouth guards should be worn with the goal of preventing dental injuries, but should be designed to include those important features (proper thickness and coverage; proper fit) which might also help stabilize the jaw and dissipate forces on impact.

REFERENCES

1. Andreasen JO. Etiology and pathogenesis of traumatic dental injuries A clinical study of 1,298 cases. Eur J Oral Sci 1970;78:329–42.
2. Kvittem B, Hardie NA, Roettger M, et al. Incidence of orofacial injuries in high school sports. J Public Health Dent 1998;58(4):288–93.
3. Yamada T, Sawaki Y, Tomida S, et al. Oral injury and mouthguard usage by athletes in Japan. Endod Dent Traumatol 1998;14(2):84–7.
4. Ljungqvist A, Jenoure PJ, Engebretsen L, et al. The International Olympic Committee (IOC) consensus statement on periodic health evaluation of elite athletes March 2009. Br J Sports Med 2009;43(9):631–43.
5. Josefsson E, Karlander EL. Traumatic injuries to permanent teeth among Swedish school children living in a rural area. Swed Dent J 1994;18(3):87–94.
6. Jeff S, Coombes PHD. Sports drinks and dental. Am J Dent 2005;18(2):101–4.
7. Flores MT, Andersson L, Andreasen JO, et al. Guidelines for the management of traumatic dental injuries. I. Fractures and luxations of permanent teeth. Dent Traumatol 2007;23:66–71.
8. Available at: http://www.dentaltraumaguide.org. Accessed January 1, 2017.

9. Kenny DJ, Barrett EJ, Casas MJ. Avulsions and intrusions: the controversial displacement injuries. J Can Dent Assoc 2003;69(5):308–13.
10. Fuselier JC, Ellis EE 3rd, Dodson TB. Do mandibular third molars alter the risk of angle fracture? J Oral Maxillofac Surg 2002;60(5):514–8.
11. Tevepaugh DB, Dodson TB. Are mandibular third molars a risk factor for angle fractures? A retrospective cohort study. J Oral Maxillofac Surg 1995;53(6):646–9.
12. Flanders RA, Bhat MJ. The incidence of orofacial injuries in sports: a pilot study in Illinois. J Am Dent Assoc 1995;126(4):491–6.
13. Hunter K. Modern mouthguards. Vol. 15, No. 3. Australia: Dental Health and Research Foundation; 1989.
14. Park JB, Shaull KL, Overton B, et al. Improving mouth guards. J Prosthet Dent 1994;72(4):373–80.
15. McCrory P. Do mouthguards prevent concussions? Br J Sports Med 2001;35: 81–2.
16. Aubry M, Meeuwisse WH, Aubry M, et al. Consensus statement on concussion in sports. Br J Sports Med 2013;47:250–8.
17. Gould TE, Piland SG, Caswell SV, et al. Preventing and managing sport-related dental and oral injuries. J Ath Tr 2016;51(10):821–39.

Index

Note: Page numbers of article titles are in **boldface** type.

A

B

C

Moving?

Make sure your subscription moves with you!

To notify us of your new address, find your **Clinics Account Number** (located on your mailing label above your name), and contact customer service at:

Email: journalscustomerservice-usa@elsevier.com

800-654-2452 (subscribers in the U.S. & Canada)
314-447-8871 (subscribers outside of the U.S. & Canada)

Fax number: 314-447-8029

Elsevier Health Sciences Division
Subscription Customer Service
3251 Riverport Lane
Maryland Heights, MO 63043

*To ensure uninterrupted delivery of your subscription, please notify us at least 4 weeks in advance of move.

ELSEVIER

Printed and bound by CPI Group (UK) Ltd, Croydon, CR0 4YY

08/05/2025

01864699-0009